Science of the Marathon
and the Art of Variable Pace Running

Véronique BILLAT, PhD ■ *Johnathan Edwards, MD*

The Science of the Marathon and the Art and Science of Variable Pace Running
Copyright © 2020
All rights reserved.
First Edition: 2020

Editor: Johnathan Edwards, M.D.
Cover: Murielle Chamarande
Formatting: Streetlight Graphics

ISBN: 978-0-9787094-2-6

No part of this book may be reproduced, scanned, or distributed in any printed or electronic form without permission. Please do not participate in or encourage piracy of copyrighted materials in violation of the author's rights. Thank you for respecting the hard work of this author.

TABLE OF CONTENTS

Foreword 1

Introduction 5

Chapter 1: Finishing a Marathon Changes Your Life Forever –
An Introduction to Variable Speed Running 13

Chapter 2: Dissecting a Marathon 19

Chapter 3: The Speed Variation of Non-Elite Marathoner Runners 31

Chapter 4: Breaking the 2-Hour Marathon and Speed Variation 41

Chapter 5: The Physiological Foundations of
Classical Endurance Training 51

Chapter 6: Increasing Your Speed Reserve 61

Chapter 7: Variable Speed Acceleration Training 78

Chapter 8: Acceleration Based Training –
Biochemistry, Enzymes, and Lactate 87

Chapter 9: Energy, Nutrition, and Human Performance 95

Chapter 10: Relationship between Speed,
VO2 max, MAS and Performance 107

Chapter 11: Critical Speed Concept 121

Chapter 12: The Real Meaning and Purpose of
Threshold Training 132

Chapter 13: Aging and Minimalistic Acceleration Training 151

Chapter 14: Listen to Your Body 162

Chapter 15: The BillaTraining Program 173

Chapter 16: Personalized Training Program
with Key Workout Sessions 185

Chapter 17: Developing your Speed Signature
for Marathon Day 201

Bibliography 209

FOREWORD

THE SCIENCE OF THE MARATHON *and the Art of Variable Pace Running* encourages you to rediscover running by gradually slowing down, running at your own pace, and learning to accelerate. In fact, it will take no longer than 30 – 40 minutes per session and 2 to 3 sessions per week. Integrating this type of training into your home or workplace is easy. This training method is equally applicable to other endurance sports like cycling, swimming, rowing, and cross-country skiing. We invite you to discover this new way of running as it is a realistic minimalist-based training using your running mind-body feelings sensations and your lifestyle.

THE AUTHORS

Véronique Billat decided to embark on a journey searching for the optimal training program for health and performance. At that time, she was a runner and international cross-country skier and trained in quantities that were often counterproductive. After completing a Doctorate in Exercise Physiology, she was able to attain a high fitness level and strike a balance between her coaching and scientific activities. The inspiration for her works (over 150 international publications and eight books) came from listening to her runners and paying attention to the fundamental problems.

In addition to her activities as a university professor, she founded the www.BillaTraining.com company to self-finance her applied research by developing training algorithms for human and animal energetics. This research takes place in real life and extreme racing situations; it does not take place on treadmills, rather in marathon races and the high mountains. It's about adapting new technologies to the needs of training and not using and analyzing them without understanding the stakes and possibilities for the improvement of human energy. Let us finally realize that human energy is the energy that increases the more we use it. It is the magical effect of running that tells us that we are alive and that we can start and progress at any age!

Johnathan Edwards is an accomplished collegiate runner, cyclist, and motocross racer. Following a brief professional motocross career, he went on to study at the University of California at Davis majoring in Physiology. After completing his medical degree in Norfolk, Virginia, he completed a year of medicine abroad in France, changing his life as he knew it. He became fluent in French and its culture. Today he lives part time in the South of France and is involved with many French organizations such as the Dakar Rally, the Ag2R La Mondial professional cycling team, the Four Days of Dunkerque professional cycling race, and the Ronde Des Sables professional motorcycle race, in Dunkerque, France. Working closely with Dr. Billat, he has mastered the www.BillaTraining.com methods for running. Dr. Edwards and Dr. Billat met because of a simple email written in French. She was intrigued that an American would write in French, and they started corresponding about sports training and nutrition. After a meeting in Paris, he enrolled in her Ph.D. program at the University of Paris. Later, she asked if he would collaborate in writing a book about running in English, and the result is *The Science of the Marathon and the Art of Variable Pace Running*.

Working closely with Dr. Billat, he has mastered the BillaTraining.com methods for running. Dr. Edwards and Dr. Billat met because of a simple email written in French. She was intrigued that an American would write in French, and they started corresponding about sports training and nutrition. After a meeting in Paris, he enrolled in her Ph.D. program at the University of Paris. Later, she asked if he would collaborate in writing a book about running in English, and the result is *The Science of the Marathon and the Art of Variable Pace Running*.

The Science of the Marathon and the Art of Variable Pace Running is about Veronique Billat's life studies and is the result of 30 years of research and practical experience. After reaching the limits of classical training for running (which is still taught in schools 30 years later), Dr. Billat decided to train in the distant hills and mountains, based upon using her sensations and abandoning the never-ending 15 sets of 200-m or four sets of 1000-m at race pace. Discovering success in her first road (Marvejols-Mende) and cross-country (Sierre-Zinal) races, she never looked back and has dedicated her life to this way of variable paced running and living.

The key to long term success without injury or overtraining is to train with quality and not quantity. This is why Dr. Billat adopted a minimalist training approach. And above all, she increased her power reserves, giving her a margin of security in very long-distance races. It is no longer necessary to train by running long distances in preparation for specific types of running races. Performance is not just about a result, but rather a road to true happiness. The practice of marathon running is, above all, a serious endeavor for anyone 10 to 100 years old, that will let you dream immense possibilities.

INTRODUCTION

IN MARATHON RUNNING, WE OFTEN hear, "above all, finish or get to the finish line!" Life is not only about racing and accepting the medal, but racing indeed adds a little spice to our lives. We must strive to perfectly integrate racing into our schedules and live life to the fullest. This book is an ode to running and racing, offering you the latest scientific innovations "put into practice." We hope to save you time and add more pleasure in running. Unnecessary miles or kilometers lead to overtraining and stress fractures. We all have the choice to run and train differently, which is not the case in our other life activities. Our minimalist training approach will get you to the finish line, feeling good, and without the mindless miles at a constant pace. The training techniques and programs in this book will give you a new second wind, and you will be able to adapt our training regimen at any age or level of performance, from beginner to elite.

If you are among those racing enthusiasts who are part of the exploding popularity of marathon running (Figure 1) or think running a marathon seems out of reach, then this book is for you! In France, female Paris marathon participants increase about 25 percent annually (half as much as in American, European, and Japanese marathons). Also, 30 percent of women who ran the Paris marathon did not even run three years ago! For example, the average age of marathon runners in the Paris Marathon is forty-one and forty years old for men and women, and the dropout rate is low (less than 5 percent for both sexes).

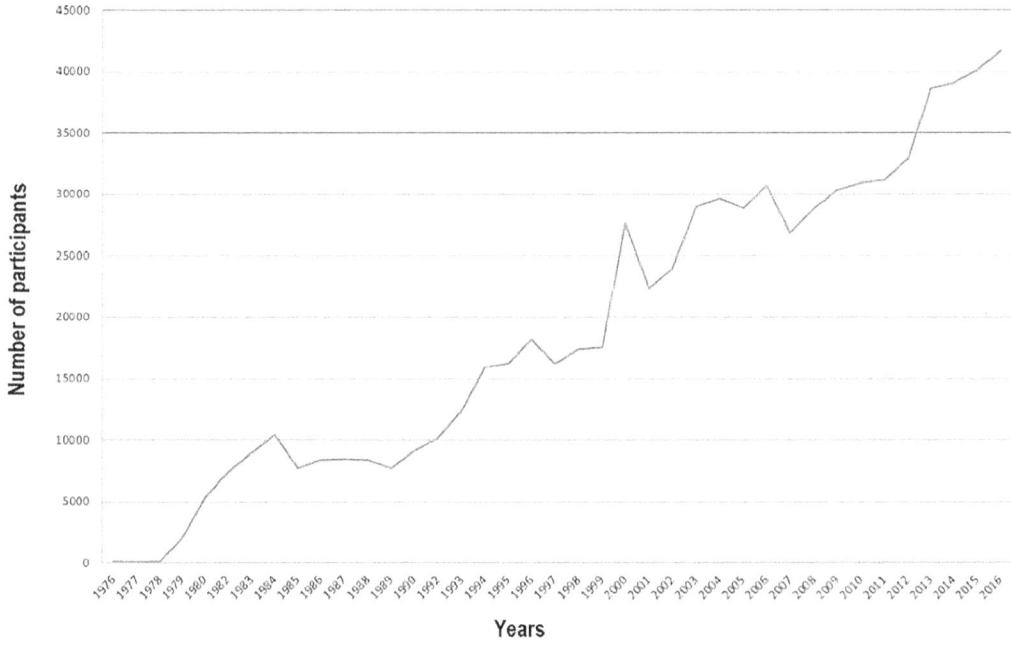

Figure 1. Evolution of the number of Paris marathon finishers from 1976 to 2016.

Before the 1970s, there were no women's distance running races in the Olympics. After the conquest of women's right to run in the early 1970s, women have had an extremely rapid growth in their participation and performance (Figure 2), which shows the significant effects of social aspects on performance. These social aspects were dominant in the early 1900s, and as the quality of life changed, it strongly influenced marathon performance in both men and women.

We can see from the graph (Figure 2) that women have had an extremely rapid growth in their marathon times, which shows the importance of social aspects on performance. Quality of life strongly influences marathon performance, which prevails at the personal level for women. The lack of consideration of social and economic factors has led to misleading predictions about the possibility of a woman running a marathon faster than a man as early as 2050 (Figure 3). An article on this subject even appeared in the prestigious journal Nature (Whipp and Ward 1992). Tabloid magazines have sensationalized articles on this subject to increase its "impact factor," contributing to the magazine ratings by the number of readers.

The Boston Marathon, the oldest in the world (124th edition in 2021), already had extraordinary growth in the number of sub-three-hour finishers' hours between 1968 and 1976. During that time, the number of marathons in the United States exploded 300 percent, and all this while women were still banned from competing!

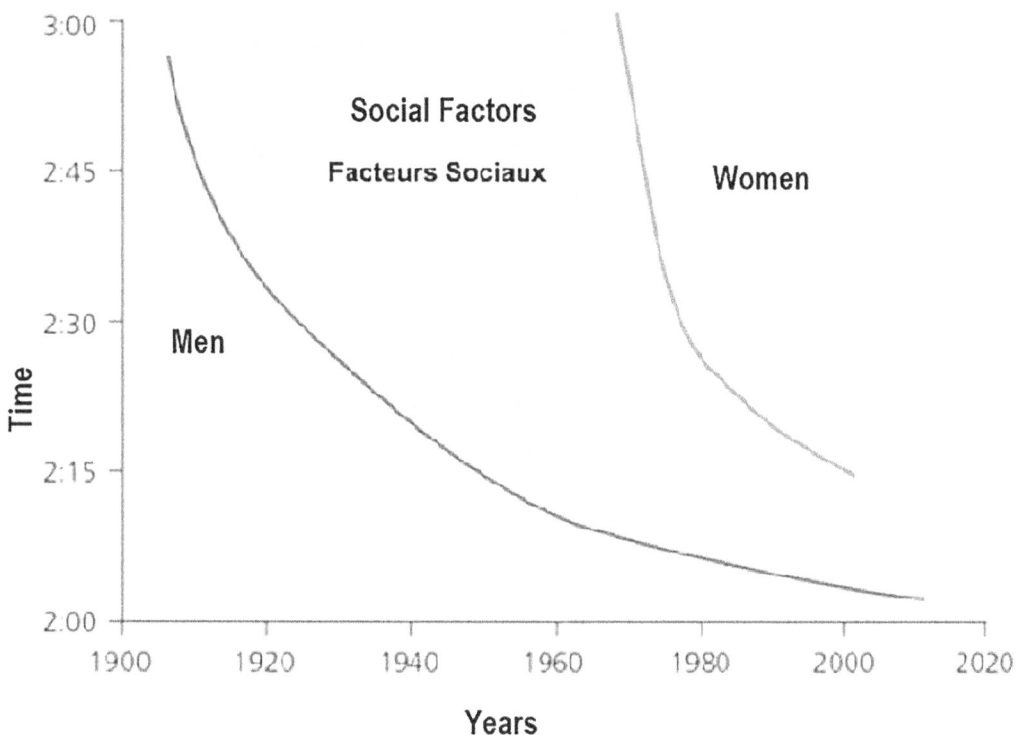

Figure 2. The evolution of the marathon records for men and women since 1900. We can see the decrease in marathon times for women was the greatest between 1984 and 1990. It was only in recent history that women could compete in marathons (Senefeld 2016). Cultural factors that lead to a difference in marathon times above 2:20 are work and professional factors and the globalization of marathon running. The differences between men and women running 2:20 and better, the most important factors are different body composition, level of hemoglobin, muscle mass, and VO2 max.

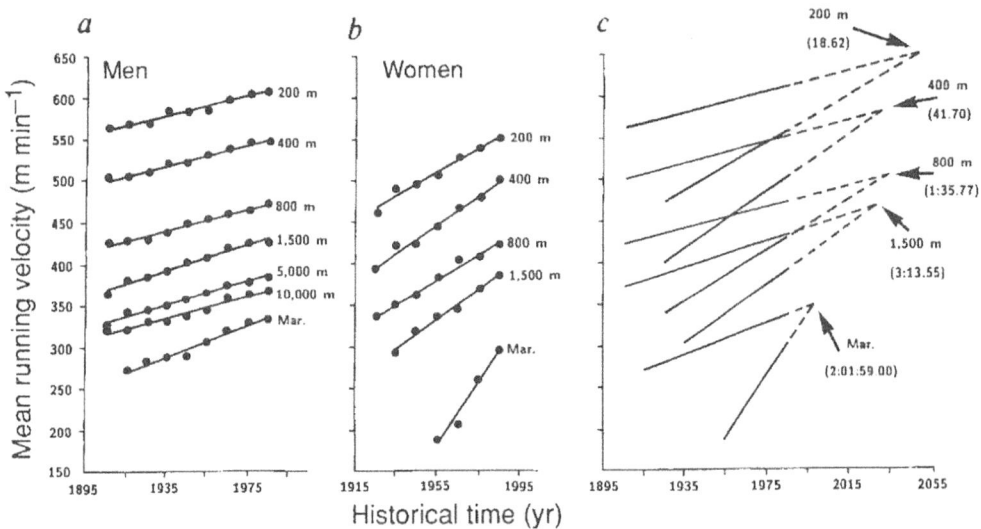

Figure 3. An extrapolative prediction of women's ability to beat men in the 1998 marathon was solely based on the rapid rise of female marathon records without considering sociological factors (Whipp and Ward 1992).

Recall the merit of Kathrine Switzer, born in 1947. She was inspired by American Roberta Louise "Bobbi" Gibb, who ran the 1966 Boston marathon in 3 hours 21 minutes and 25 seconds without being officially entered into the race. Kathrine Switzer asked her university cross-country coach to let her run the marathon with him. Her coach refused, stating that a woman was not "tough enough" to run a marathon and that this could lead to her "uterus falling out or masculinization." She convinced him nevertheless by running distances greater than the marathon. Switzer entered the 1967 Boston Marathon and was granted a number as no rules existed stipulating that women could not compete. It is said that Switzer was issued a number through an "oversight" in the entry screening process. She started the Boston Marathon, even though the "official rules" prohibited women from participating and was treated as a trespasser when the error was discovered. On the day of the race, she was encouraged by the other participants to continue, but at the fourth mile, the race organizer (Jock Semple) attempted to remove her from the race. She was heroically defended by her coach and other runners and finished in 4 hours and 20 minutes, one hour more than her hero Bobbi Gibb. Following her race, Kathrine Switzer was disqualified and suspended by the American Athletics Federation, losing her right to compete. The organization explicitly forbade women from participating in any competition with male runners. Switzer then campaigned the Boston Athletic Association to allow women to participate in the marathon and for the women's marathon to be part of the Olympics. In 1972, the Boston Marathon was officially opened to women. In 1984, the first Olympic women's marathon in Los Angeles took place. It was won in 2 hours 24 minutes and 52 seconds (an incredible time) by an American runner Joan Benoit (*Chaffee, K. Her Fearless Run: Kathrine Switzer's Historic Boston Marathon, 2019*).

Switzer won the New York Marathon in 1974 with a time of 3 hours 7 minutes and 29 seconds (59th overall). She competed in a total of thirty-five marathons, and her best time was 2 hours 51 minutes and 37 seconds (Boston 1975). In 2017, fifty years after her first participation, she participated in the Boston Marathon, with the same bib number "261" as in 1967 and finished the race in 4 hours 44 minutes and 31 seconds. The current women's marathon record is 2 hours and 15 minutes, only 11 percent slower than the fastest male runner. Even more impressive is that the average difference between mid-pack male and female runners (over 4 hours and 6 minutes) is 30 minutes, which is also 11 percent.

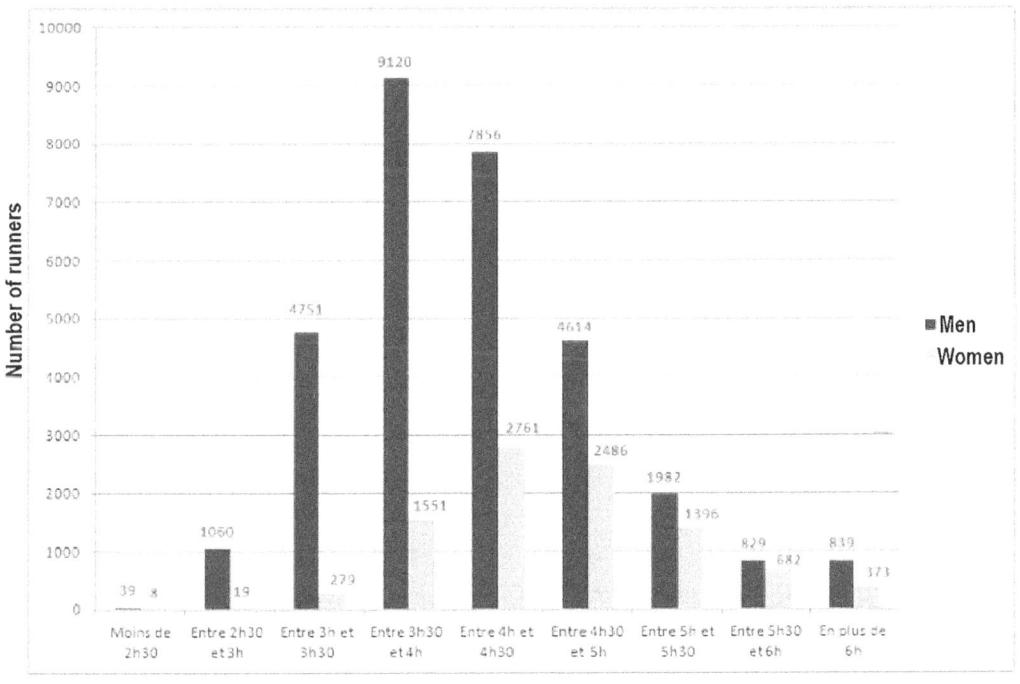

Figure 4. Breakdown of chronometric times of the men and women runners of the 2015 Paris Marathon.

The distribution of performances between males and females is shifted by 30 minutes, which tells us about the differences in marathon performance between the two sexes (Figure 4). India (the second largest country in terms of population) has finally seen an emergence of running events. Indeed, in India, where endurance sports are poorly represented, the recent success of running events is surprising. Organized events are based upon the European model, with their modes of communication, promotion, and event leadership. But the Indians have made running into their own by giving it a symbolic dimension and celebration. For example, in modern globalized cities in India, like Bangalore, the demand is so strong that every weekend several races are organized and bring together thousands of runners. In 2014, more than twenty-three thousand runners, sometimes running in saree, sandals or even barefoot, and wearing denim, took part in a race, sponsored by the consulting giant Tata Consultancy Services. The competition was also sponsored by the big western multinationals like Nike, BMW, DHL, etc. Carl Lewis, a running legend, gave the official start, and the winners received nearly one million dollars. The major international brands have understood the benefits of sponsoring these events, and the practice of "naming" these events has become widespread in India.

For instance, the Mumbai Marathon became the Standard Chartered Mumbai Marathon, named after a bank. The Delhi Half Marathon or the Airtel Delhi Half Marathon is named after a telephone company. This economic aspect of running favors mass participation and attracts many elite runners from other countries. This contributes not only to the fall of records but also inflating the price of the race entries. The registration cost represents a significant portion of the median annual salary of a running competitor in India, which is about 600 dollars. For example, this budget could be divided into four major categories: 34 percent for shoes, 26 percent for registration fees, 21 percent for fabrics, and 19 percent for accessories (especially digital). These mass races attract sponsors, who, in turn, increase the race offerings favoring this explosion of organized events.

Many in the running community are focused on records, for example, breaking the 2-hour marathon. Running records are not just about physiology. We can, therefore, conclude that the marathon record is about physiological factors, but it also has to do with environmental, social, and economic factors. Beyond the world record, beyond 2-hours, this book is interested in your performance!

Finally, we understand that many of the principles outlined in this book are advanced, even for many running coaches. But the principles that you will learn in this book will change how you train and think about the marathon and life!

CHAPTER 1

FINISHING A MARATHON CHANGES YOUR LIFE FOREVER – AN INTRODUCTION TO VARIABLE SPEED RUNNING

THE REWARDS OF MARATHON RUNNING are that of a different kind, difficult to define, but none the less real. Running is a great way to get fit, feel better, and form new relationships. Not many things are so simple in life that with a pair of shoes, shorts, and the willingness to move a little or a lot, the satisfaction of running is unparalleled. Marathon running is the only sport that gives you a chance to run against the best in the world by paying for the entry. It is hard to believe that eighteen men lined up at the start of the first Olympic marathon on April 10, 1896, in Greece. A century before, people's attitude toward running was quite different. Running was the most efficient means of relaying messages mostly for wealthy people and governments. A paradigm shift happened, and humans started to take up running for pleasure. Today, more than 2 million people take up running each year, and all of them hoping to find one thing, change.

Contrary to popular belief, running and training for a marathon can be fun. The training involved with a marathon absorbs a lot of time, especially for those of us with full-time jobs or a family. Many runners spend more than three-hundred hours per year training for a marathon. Considering the cost of entry fees, equipment, and traveling, marathon running is certainly not profitable. So why do we do it? Running is about many things, but it's mainly about transformation. It often happens when a person recognizes that they are getting older and desire better health; the decision to run a marathon is a step towards this goal. Most people are not born to run; we are either too short, too tall, overweight, or not athletic, yet our disadvantages are part of the very transformation that we seek from running. Running makes us aware of our body and nature itself, and we emerge with a clearer perspective of the person we genuinely want to become. The chances are that you are not genetically gifted with the body of a fitness model, and it is highly unlikely that running will ever transform you into one. But what running can do is to help transform you into your ideal self, perhaps who you think you should be in life. Often in our forties, it follows a doctor's visit or family illness, and you panic feeling like you are going to die early. Running is about the transformation from darkness back into the light. People gravitate towards running to be healthy and happy.

IT'S ABOUT THE JOURNEY

People new to running approach their first marathon with some amount of trepidation and fear, along with transforming hope. It is the journey that changes the person. Runners take care of each other through uninhibited encouragement. It helps if you can run a distance between three and six miles and have some base fitness. If you come from another sport, you will find the training easier than someone who is starting from the couch. There are many ways to run a marathon as it is as much of an art as a science. Many runners choose a single distance and run it at the same monotonous pace because that is what we have been taught. Several popular running books tell you to start slow, stay at one pace, and finish fast! Humans were never designed to run at just one pace. In the running world, we call these "one pace wonders." Certainly, running this way results in increased fitness and gratification, but ultimately leads to fitness plateaus, boring and stale workouts, loss of motivation, and injury. Humans instinctually vary the pace, and if we let it happen naturally, we can run for a lifetime and enjoy it.

Dr. Veronique Billat a French physiologist, and researcher, has dedicated her life to the physiology of running and endurance training. She earned her PhD. from the University of Grenoble in France and is a full professor at the University of Paris. She is among the most published sports physiologists of our time and is truly a leader in the science of individualized training for health and performance. She has written several books about running. Our goal is to show you that there is another way to run, without stress, injuries, huge time commitments, and naturally. In 2016, she gave a TED talk on this subject in Lille, France. Her Paris laboratory, just north of the Place de la Republique, is known for its canals, bustling streets, excellent restaurants, and French markets. Dr. Billat's innovative research changes the way we run and train for the marathon and any distance for that matter. A competitive athlete herself with a one hour and eighteen minutes personal best (PB) for the half-marathon, she has coached many amateur and professional runners to a personal record (PR), Boston Qualifier (BQ), and to the finish line. Veronique's more than thirty years of research focuses on identifying high-quality workouts and optimal long-term training programs. Above all else, her training methods are extremely practical, and you can literally take her research and run with it.

Most runners do better with a training plan, but buyer beware. Many training plans take you from the couch to the marathon in a prescribed number of weeks using a long-slow-distance (LSD) approach of gradual mileage progression. Most training plans neglect how to tap into the innate running potential that we all possess. Whether you are a "weekend marathoner" (in French we say, Le Marathonier du Dimanche) or a professional athlete, the training techniques outlined in this book will help you. Many concepts in this book are advanced, but we try to present them in an easy to understand format and every runner will gain insight. Dr. Billat has put her life's work into these concepts, and most importantly she has the time, studies, and results to prove these training techniques work towards your success and importantly running naturally and injury free.

Key questions to ask yourself are, "why do I need a coach?" We all need a coach, otherwise, you are limiting your success. A good coach can see the things you are blind to; they watch how you run, analyze your times and technique, ultimately giving you the athlete, an optimized perspective of your goals. Good coaches create a safe environment so that you can see yourself more clearly, build structure and accountability, identify blind spots in a training program, add clarity to your goals, stay on track, gain a competitive advantage, and stoke your success. A coach gives the athlete confidence to reach levels of performance that may not have been possible otherwise. At www.BillaTraining.com, we are here to coach you to your running and marathon success. This book is just the first step.

Perhaps the hardest thing to teach runners is that more is not better, and that marathon running does not have to be hard. There is perpetual controversy in the elite circles of running of whether high mileage or high intensity is better for optimal results. If you are not an elite runner, then this controversy may not be particularly important to you. Changing up your routine is more important than following a fixed "scientific" plan. In life, plans change (travel, health, work, etc.), but the body naturally adapts to routines. To progress, it is important to change things up. Even if you don't care about VO2 max or maximal aerobic speed (MAS), the ideas you learn will stay with you for life and keep you running, and most of all, loving to run. Running is an endless source of learning, especially if you listen to your body.

VARIABLE PACED RUNNING

Varying the speed or pace you run at is exactly the opposite of running at a constant pace or the same speed. It sounds easy enough, but most runners, whether at a club or school, are taught to run at a target pace and little else. Variation of speeds while running is not only natural, but it is healthier for you. For now, leave your watch on the table and let's rediscover the real art of running!

Many factors affect the runner during endurance events, such as altitude, changes in terrain, fatigue, elevation, health, hydration, nutrition, temperature, and more. A runner may strategize to maintain a target pace to achieve a particular result. Understanding how and why we need to have variability in our running speeds leads to a better knowledge of the factors influencing our marathon performance. This helps the runner to complete a marathon successfully and improve race performance. An intriguing aspect of varying the pace is that homeostasis is maintained, that is, you will never come close to cracking or bonking, especially at that mythic twenty-third mile. When the wrong pace is chosen and followed, several things are sure to happen – cramps, fatigue, slowing of the pace, and the inability to finish the marathon. Most marathon training programs target maintaining a specific pace for 26.2 miles. If you are interested in finishing a marathon in a decent time and feeling good at the end, that is, after the twenty-third mile, then variable speed running is one of the most important techniques you will learn. Furthermore, variable pace running keeps it fun and enjoyable. The best runners have a strong mind-body connection and learn to run by feel. Running by feel is not as straightforward as it sounds, it takes practice, but the result is well worth it.

> ## A Tale of Two Marathon Runners
>
> ### Marathon runner example: Joe
>
> Joe is a forty-two-year-old office worker who decided to change his life and run his first marathon. Joe started his training using a traditional coach who prescribes a program from the couch to running a marathon in eighteen weeks. Initially, Joe begins running slowly, and is told to increase his mileage gradually, always at the same pace. Joe does great and loves the idea of running and progressively builds his mileage, but always at a prescribed monotonous pace. Joe's coach has him running just about every day and gives him certain distance and pace goals each week leading up to the marathon. Halfway through the program, Joe has lost weight, feeling better, but now has a mild nagging knee injury that causes pain at the end of a 10-mile run. The coach tells Joe that he needs to test his newfound fitness in a half-marathon. Reluctantly, Joe starts the half-marathon and finishes the race in a respectable time. However, he can now really feel his knee pain. Two days later, Joe cannot run, as it is too painful. Joe sees his doctor and finds out that he cannot run for several weeks and may not even be able to compete in the marathon.
>
> ### Marathon runner example two: Cindy
>
> Cindy is a forty-two-year-old office worker and has been thinking about changing her life for some time now. After some reflection, she decides to enter a marathon. She signs up with BillaTraining.com as she likes the idea of running to her sensations and the minimalistic training program. Cindy performs the initial steps on the website and submits her RABIT test. Through her coach at BillaTraining.com, she starts a running program. Cindy learns what it means to run according to her sensations and using variable-based accelerations. She is taught to run at different intensities, using easy, medium, hard, and sprint, and often without a watch. She trains 3 – 4 times per week. Her marathon plan is to start fast, then slow down below her established average pace, and then finish fast. On the day of her marathon, everything went according to plan and she noticed

> that she still had plenty of energy at the twentieth mile while everyone around her was struggling to finish. Cindy was transformed after her first marathon and went on to complete several more.

Together we will take a closer look at some world-class marathon runners and dissect what happened in their races. We will also outline the strategy for breaking the two-hour marathon and how it can be done by varying the pace. With the evolution of science, technology, and the Internet, we have been able to analyze PRs and highlight the factors leading to these results. Most PRs began with a fast start, then a decrease in speed, variations in speed, and finally, a fast finish. This book provides the practice and theory allowing you to discover variable pace running and gain confidence (even discovering it). The marathon is too often thought of as a burden (even if one denies it), instead it should give us daily astonishment in the way it transforms our lives!

CHAPTER ONE SUMMARY

CONCEPT: Varying the speed or pace you run at is exactly the opposite of running at a constant pace or the same speed. An intriguing aspect of varying the pace is that homeostasis is maintained, that is, you will never come close to cracking or bonking, especially at that mythic twenty-third mile. When the wrong pace is chosen and followed, several things are sure to happen – the resulting cramps, fatigue, slowing of pace, and not being able to finish the marathon. Understanding how and why we need to have variability in our running speeds leads to a better knowledge of the factors influencing our marathon performance. This helps the runner to complete a marathon successfully and improve race performance.

APPLICATION: Variation of speeds while running is natural, and it is healthier for you. For now, leave your watch on the table and let's rediscover the true art of running! Most marathon training programs target maintaining a specific pace for 26.2 miles. For runners interested in finishing a marathon in a decent time and feeling good at the end, that is, after the twenty-third mile, variability of pace is one of the most essential running techniques you will learn.

CHAPTER 2

DISSECTING A MARATHON

A MARATHON IS MORE THAN JUST running 26.2 miles or 42.2 kilometers. Taking a closer look or "dissecting" your marathon and training runs is a tool that ensures the training and effort is a success. Learning to dissect your running performances establishes running ability, aerobic profiles, running intensities, and strategy. Examining a race performance can indicate where your brain says no more, but the legs still have it. Unfortunately, most runners only resort to analyzing the details of their performance after a bad event. Many people are eager to tell you why you ran poorly in a race, whether it be strategy, fuel, heat exhaustion, or bad running economy. But none of it matters unless you take a more-in-depth look into what happened during that run. At the BillaTraining.com headquarters, we have a team dedicated to dissecting running performances.

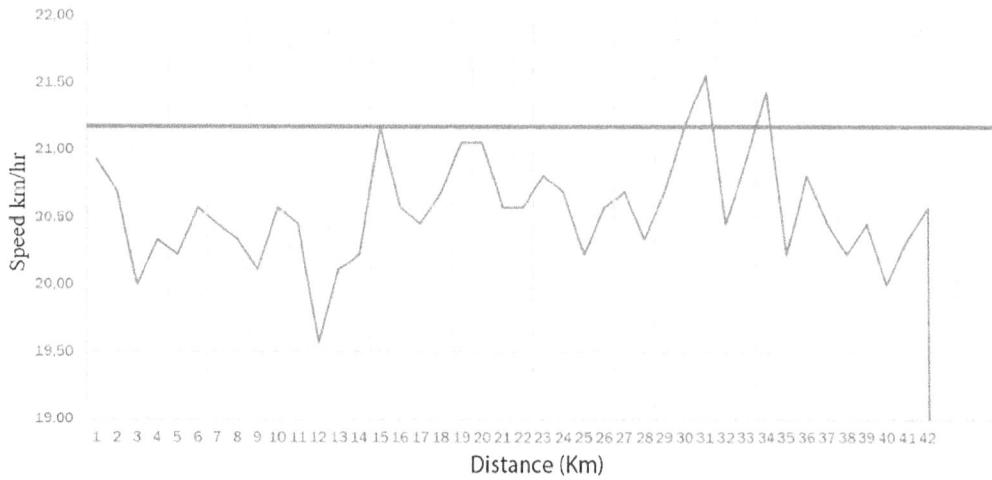

Figure 5. Analysis of the world marathon record of Dennis Kimetto in Berlin (2014) detailed over 1-kilometer intervals.

DISSECTING A WORLD RECORD MARATHON PERFORMANCE

Dennis Kimetto's 2014 marathon performance in Berlin (Figure 5) is important because it shows a world record marathon performance over 1-km intervals, the only ones we currently have. The red horizontal line represents the speed bar for the sub-2-hour marathon. Looking closer in Figure 5, we can see that, Kimetto started very quickly for 1 km and then slowed down during his world record attempt. Then he ran in a varying or oscillating pattern, accelerating to more than a 2:42 minute/km or a 4:49 minute/mile pace towards the end and then finishing below his average speed. At the thirty-first and thirty-fourth kilometers, his speed was on par for a sub-2-hour marathon. Further analysis reveals speed variations of 10 – 15 percent of his average speed (in km/min).

It is interesting to look at the relative speed variations in elite male runners in several marathons (Figure 6); the top three finishers consistently show a convex-shaped (U-shaped) curve in their race from start to finish, whereas the rest have a clear linear downward trend. When we look at the elite women, they show a concave-type curve (peaking about the twenty-fifth or thirty-fifth km). The only exception was in the Athens Olympics, where the top elite women ran a convex curve like the men. These convex and concave curves are essential because there are specific reasons for these patterns. For example, there was much more at stake in the women's races than to simply run a fast time. The winners of an Olympic marathon are well compensated. In the Athens marathon, the heat was a factor, but even that did not slow them down. Even more, we do not observe a systematic correlation among the runners before the thirtieth kilometer. The rewards of a race often dictate how it will play out and the variation in speeds observed. In the elite men, the field is dense, the competition is fierce, and the pacers (rabbits) strongly affect the dynamics of the race. In contrast, pacers are seldom used in women's races. Looking at the world record run in Berlin, the winner led the race from the fifth kilometer!

AN INTERESTING ANECDOTE OF 1000 METERS:

A 2001 study of the best marathon runners of all time including former European marathon record holder Antonio Pinto *(2h06min36s) in 2001 and Norwegian Sondre Nordstad Moen (2h05min48s) looked at the difference between the two groups of marathoners: those who ran a time between

2h06min to 2h11min and another group who ran 2h12min to 2h16min. **It was only a difference of 1000-m in a 10-km section of the marathon that dictated the difference between the two groups** (Billat 2001).

Another study looked at the times of the first fifty finishers of the 2007 and 2008 Berlin Marathons (world record of Haile Gebrselassie). It showed that the first three finishers ran a "U-shaped pattern," meaning that they started quickly, slowed down, and near the end, they accelerated to about the same pace at which they started. The runners' race strategy was to economize their times (using a pacer until the half-marathon point). Based on the experience of the individual runner and using the memory of the pain sensations as the distance accrued, the runner will accelerate in a precise manner (*feed-forward mechanism), which is similar to "dosing the effort." If this dose of effort turns out to be too painful, the runner will back off slightly and continue with that pace. The feed-forward mechanism is important because the goal is to limit the neural or central drive to the muscles. The electromyographic (EMG) activity is submaximal when an individual is making a peak voluntary effort, the muscles still have the capability. The physiological signals of the feed-forward mechanism appear to come from the brain, specifically the hypothalamus. During this time, the gap between expected and experienced pain can induce a change in stride frequency, reducing the propulsive forces compensated by a longer heel strike time. If the pace becomes unbearable, the speed will drop or even decrease to walking speed or zero. Twenty-five percent of runners competing in Olympic marathons do not finish the race. This percentage is higher than the dropout rate in the Paris Marathon, where there are more than fifty thousand runners! The dropout rate was similar for men and women, about 15 percent. One reason there is such a high dropout in the Olympic races is primarily economic. Once a runner knows that he/she will not place well in the Olympic marathon, they pull-out to keep their body "fresh" for future races where they will have a chance to earn prize money. Professional runners must be careful about over-racing their bodies to the point that they are "burned out" for the rest of the season. Keep in mind that the Olympic marathon is in the summer, the Boston marathon is in the spring, and the New York marathon is in the fall.

*Feed-forward regulation limits central drive to the muscles so that EMG activity is submaximal when an individual is making a peak voluntary effort.

Science of the Marathon

* 2h06min36s is written as two hours six minutes and thirty-six seconds.

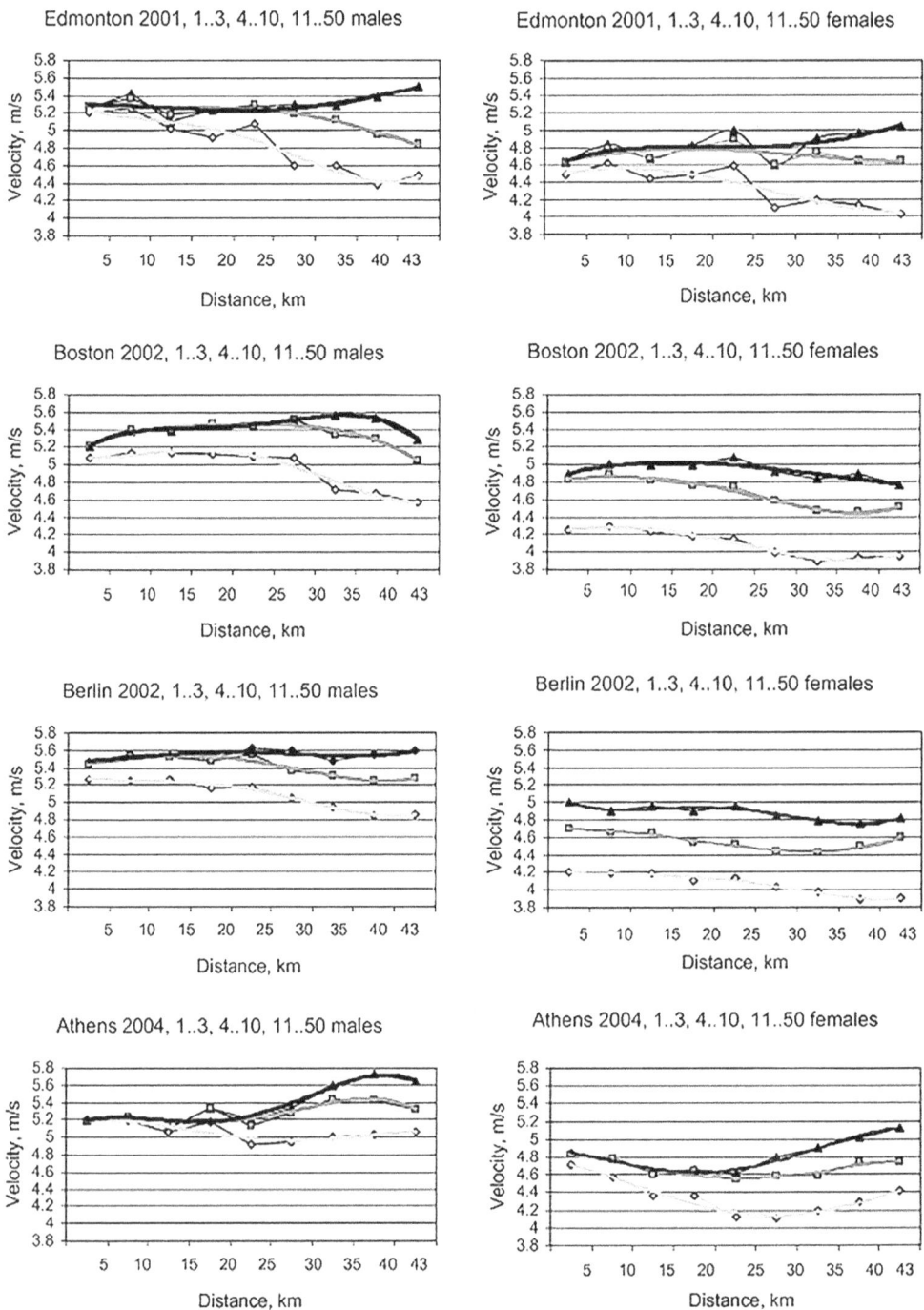

Figure 6. The average running speed per distance interval of 5 km for the first ten men and women (triangle, black and wide line and thin for men and women) and the next 40 (square light gray and dark gray line for men on the left and women on the right) (Erdmann and Lipinska 2013).

THE IMPORTANCE OF A U-SHAPED CURVE

One of the many benefits of practicing variation of speeds while running is that it allows the runner to tolerate a more considerable increase in body temperature than if they were running at a constant pace; thus supporting the notion that the upper limits of temperature regulation are modifiable (Marino 2012). Running at constant speeds adds more stress and muscle fatigue, which will become more evident.

The speed of a marathon follows a downward trend about every 10-km. Gebrselassie during the Dubai Marathon, as well as the top fifty finishers of the Berlin Marathon, clearly show this trend. We can see this by analyzing the runner's times every 5-km, and the trend becomes more oscillating every 1-km. Also, within each 10-km segment, Gebrselassie stabilizes his effort by oscillating his speeds up and down. These drops in speed are more pronounced in less efficient runners.

Women runners seem to employ more cautious strategies in their speed management due to greater anticipation of expected pain as compared to the pain they experience during the race. In general, women have an increased tolerance to pain concerning the effort they put out in relation to their physiology. In many cases, professional women endurance athletes have a speed zone that is felt and calibrated according to their perception as being "easy," when in fact it is medium or even hard when we look at the physiology. They do not run faster when their perception is medium or hard, instead their oxygen consumption peaks.

A large reserve of speed is essential for an elite runner because it allows for a fast start and the ability to oscillate his/her speed and recover during the race. The best race strategy for setting PBs and world records is to run in a convex-type pattern (U-shaped curve). World record runner, Haile Gebrselassie adopted precisely this strategy. One reason this strategy works is because a fast start makes it possible to get ahead of the target time while the legs are fresh early in the race and then in the later parts of the race, being able to accelerate. Any runner can adopt this type of strategy with enough training. We have consistently highlighted that even with a modest speed reserve, this convex curve running strategy is essential to avoid early fatigue or bonking. This alternating pace strategy allows the runner to run less above his average pace and more below his average pace. Thus, the adage, "slow down, and you'll go faster!"

By this point, everything seems academic and the concepts of variable and oscillating speeds, absolute values, and speed reserves seem confusing. But have patience and these concepts will become clear later in the book.

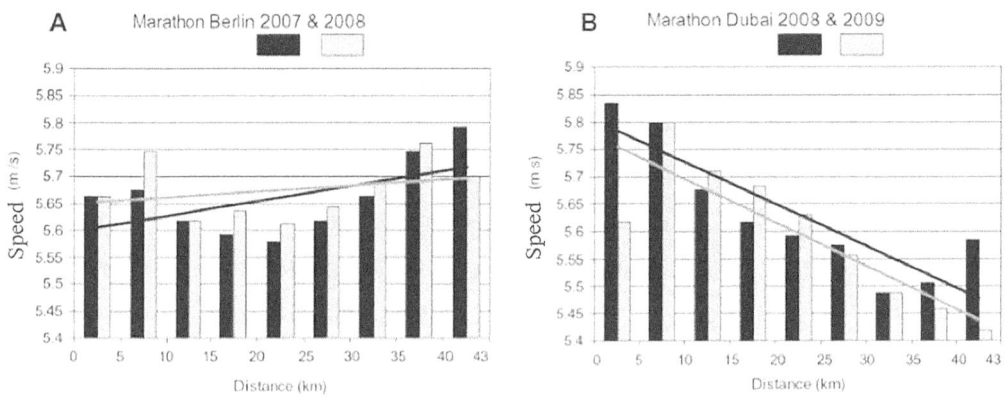

Figure 7. Haile Gebrselassie's speed variations in Berlin and Dubai during the 2008 and 2009 editions. Successful U-race (A) in Berlin by Haile Gebrselassie compared to the failed one (B) during his world record attempt at Dubai.

We see in Figure 7 that the U (convex) speed curve (Berlin) of the world marathon record holder Gebrselassie differs from the descending slope (Dubai). The drop in speeds in the Dubai Marathon may be due to the fact the race is held in January when it is hot, whereas the Berlin Marathon is cooler and held in September. The Dubai race reveals a concave shape when you look at the speeds. This is typical of a slow-starting race with an attempt to regain the time by accelerating at the halfway point. The problem with this strategy is the runner is less resistant to fatigue during the race. Running in a U-shaped curve allows you to spend more time below your average pace. Again, this is achieved by a fast start, then slowing down below your average pace, and finally accelerating well above your average pace near the end. Your speed reserves should be sufficient so that you do not have to run a very long time at your target pace, otherwise you will probably find yourself cracking after the halfway point because you wanted to ensure that you did not "fall behind" your target pace. This is why you must dare to run above your target speed during the start and finish of a marathon!

WHY VARIABLE PACE RUNNING IS BETTER

Many runners try to maintain a constant pace that is too fast. When a runner attempts to hold an overly ambitious target pace, this results in fatigue and "cracking," and inevitably leads to an average pace much below the runner's goal. An example of this is shown in Figure 10. There is a drastic fall below the target pace because the runner's average pace is set too high. It is important to stress that maintaining a specific target pace is difficult to achieve compared to "running to feel" during a race. Several reasons exist why variable paced running is advantageous: temperature, lactate, and glycogen. Heat is better regulated when running a variable versus a constant pace (Marino 2012). By varying your pace, lactate equilibrium is maintained allowing, the body to have a reserve of energy. Furthermore, holding a constant pace is difficult because lactate is continuously building and not being recycled, especially later in a marathon. In the heart and muscle cells, lactate is used for fuel as it is incorporated into the Krebs cycle. Achieving a high equilibrium of lactate (above 4 mmol) and having a good energy reserve while running a marathon, is the goal. We often observe lactate levels reaching up into the 8 mmol/L range! Another downside to constant pace running is that the body uses glycogen early, leading to an inevitable decrease in performance around the halfway mark. We propose a fast start for about 1-2 km, which does not significantly deplete glycogen stores. Most runners start to lose energy about 1 hour and 4 minutes into a marathon.

Modeling speeds for a world record (marathon) for men and women shows that the negative split (a faster second part of the race than the first) is an important factor for success. A convex-shaped curve is more in line with the physiological reality of a fast start strategy, followed by a "letting go," and accelerating from the 30 km point. Maintaining a constant target pace is extremely risky, hence why we teach the strategy of varying the speed according to your sensations and considering your metabolic capabilities. Learning to run according to your sensations does not happen all at once and takes practice. To better understand this concept of varying the speed, we can dissect the race into 1-km segments. This shows us how a runner attempts to preserve his/her ergonomics and energy produced over a time interval (in joules × seconds), which amounts to stabilizing the speed over a short distance. This principle of "stability of action" or "least action" was discovered by the great physicist and mathematician Pierre Maupertuis. Understanding the laws of "least action" allows us to better understand the physical principles regulating the speed/stroke distance.

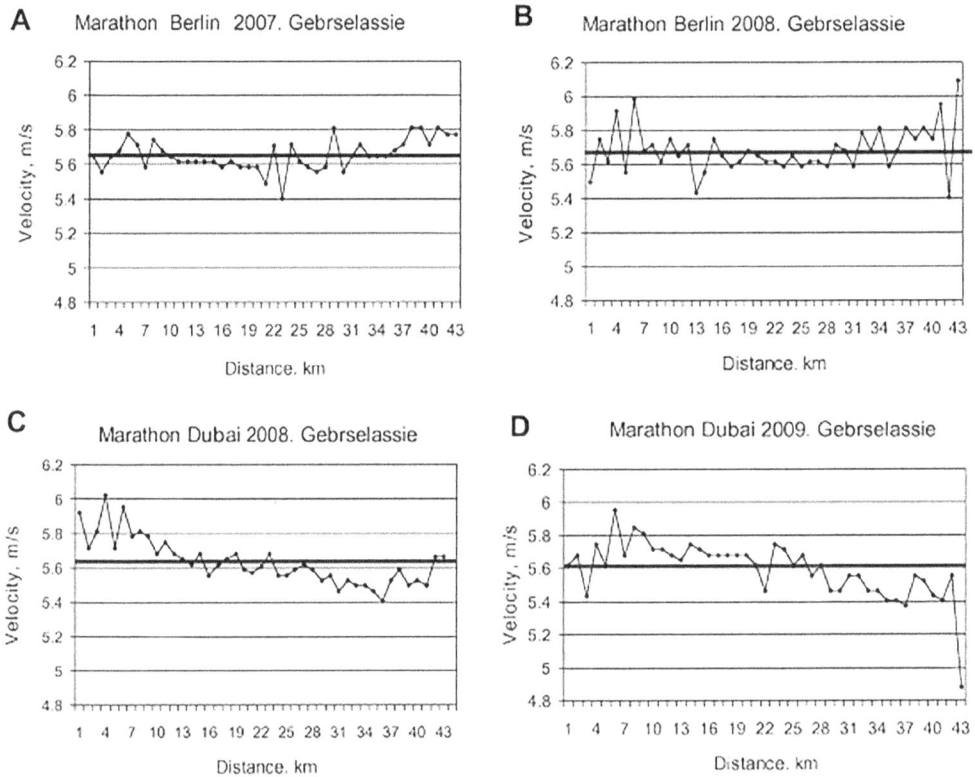

Figure 8. Halile Gebrselassie's speed measured every kilometer (fine line) at the 2008 and 2009 editions of the Berlin and Dubai Marathons. We can see that in the "failed" races in Dubai, Haile ran more in his higher speeds than his average speeds (bold line), and the distances ran below the average were well below that which explained the final result (Erdmann and Lipinska 2013).

Indeed, the best runners spend more time below their average running pace than average runners. We use simple statistics to break the run into numbers and graphs. For example, if you have a race where the distribution of your pace is towards the right, you have optimized your performance and your average pace will be higher than your median. This can be seen by the asymmetry of the running speed histogram in Figure 9. The median pace is that speed over which you ran the most distance during your marathon, while the average is the distance of the marathon divided by your chronometric time at the finish line. Another way to think about running below your average pace, is to run with the goal of being "relaxed" and efficient. This results in your average pace being higher than your median.

> ## Statistical Concepts – A Refresher
>
> **Statistics are essential for analyzing running times and performances.**
>
> Mean, median, and mode are the main measures of a statistical series. They serve to analyze a set of small numbers using "characteristic" values.
>
> - Average: The "average" value is equal to the sum of all values in the series divided by the total. For example: The average of the series $\{1, 2, 3, 4, 5, 6, 7\}$ is $(1 + 2 + 3 + 4 + 5 + 6 + 7) / 7 = 28/7 = 4$.
>
> - Median: The median of a set of values (sample, population …) is a value x, which makes it possible to cut the set of values into two equal parts: on one side, 50 percent of the values, which are all lower or equal to x, and on the other side, the other 50 percent of the values, all of which are greater than or equal to x. Example: The median of the series $\{1, 4, 12, 21, 40, 50, 55\}$ is 21 because there are as many values as or less than 21 than values greater than or equal to 21.
>
> - Mode: The mode, or dominant value, is the most represented value of any variable in a given population. For example, the mode of the series $\{3, 5, 7, 5, 8, 3, 5, 9, 5, 1, 5\}$ is 5 because it appears three times, the largest occurrence.

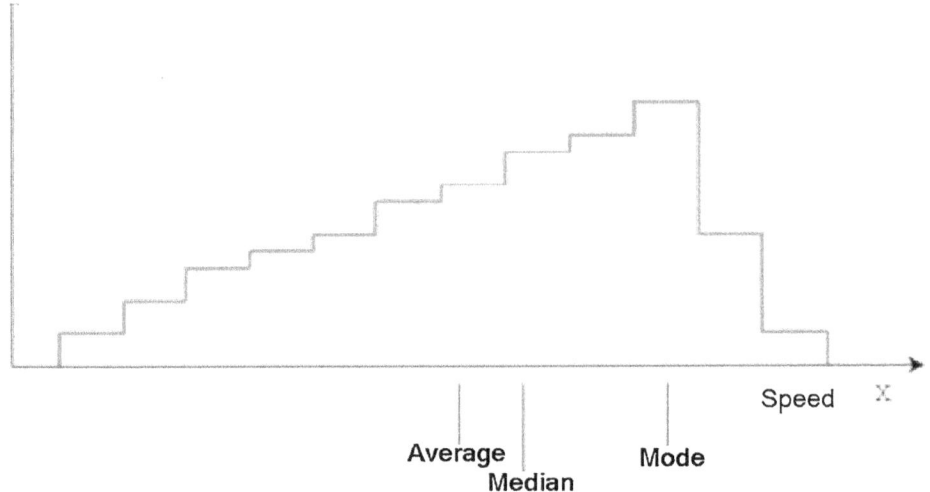

Figure 9. Histogram of running speeds during a marathon. A successful race is run more frequently below its final average speed (since the median is below average). This means that we have a "positive" asymmetry. The mode is the speed at which you ran the longest.

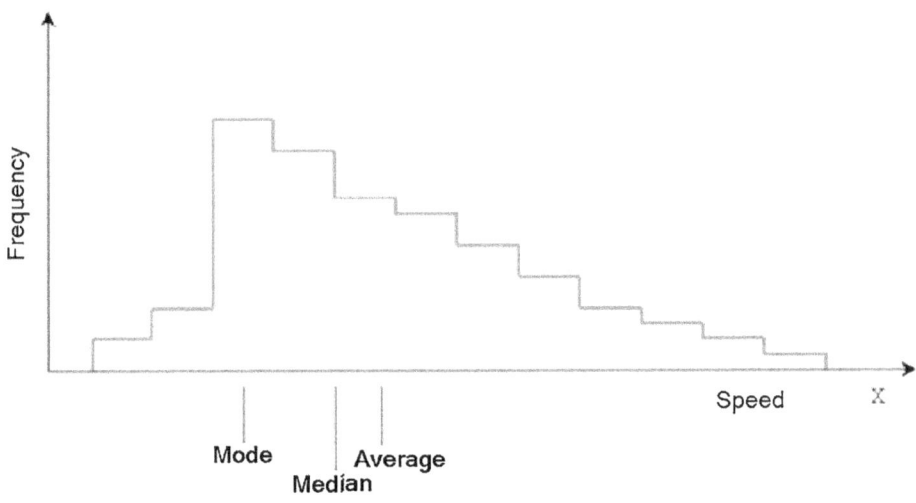

Figure 10. Histogram of running speeds during a marathon. A failed race is when a runner spent more time above the final average speed (since the median is greater than the average). We then have a so-called "negative" asymmetry, and the asymmetry coefficient is positive.

There is no point in running above your average pace, until you learn to start fast and then immediately slow down to get into a comfort zone with a large margin of safety. It takes a lot of training and practice to be able to run above your average pace. On the contrary, a failed race is one where a runner tries to hold a certain target pace and ends up cracking before the end. When this occurs, it usually means that we ran most of the marathon at a pace above the average, and as a result, the median pace is higher than the average pace (Figure 10). By analyzing your marathon, you can visualize this distribution of speeds and look for ways to improve. It is important to neglect the extreme values (GPS artifact, prolonged stops at a station, or accidents). The marathon truly is something that resists us, yet we gain so much enjoyment from its accomplishments as it is both predictable, yet so unpredictable.

CHAPTER TWO SUMMARY

CONCEPT: Observing the relative variations in speed in elite male marathon runners, the top three finishers consistently show a convex shaped (U-shaped) curve in their race from start to finish. The rest have a clear linear downward trend. When we look at the elite women, they show a concave-type curve (peaking about the twenty-fifth or thirty-fifth km). These convex and concave curves are important because there are specific reasons for these patterns. In the women's races, there was much more at stake for them than to simply run a fast time as measured by the stopwatch. In the elite men's field, the field is dense, competition is fierce and importantly the existence of pacers (rabbits) strongly affects how the race is ran. In contrast, pacers are rarely used in women's races. Looking at the world record run in Berlin, the winner led the race from the fifth kilometer!

APPLICATION: The Importance of a U-Shaped Curve is one of the many benefits of practicing variation of running speeds. It allows the runner to tolerate greater increases in body temperature and lactate concentrations than if they were running at a constant pace. This supports the notion that the upper limits of temperature regulation are modifiable. Running at constant speeds adds more stress and muscle fatigue, and not the temperature increases per se. The best race strategy for setting PBs and world records is to run in a convex-type pattern (U-shaped curve). Any runner can adopt this type of strategy with enough training. Indeed, we have consistently highlighted that even with a modest speed reserve, this convex curve running strategy is essential in avoiding early fatigue or bonking. In addition, this alternating pace strategy allows the runner to run less above his average pace and more below his average pace. Thus, the adage, "slow down and you'll go faster!"

CHAPTER 3
THE SPEED VARIATION OF NON-ELITE MARATHONER RUNNERS

A good strategy for success in a world record marathon is a U-shaped race pattern. It can be the difference between a successful elite runner setting a world record or PB, versus that of a failed race. You might be thinking that speed variation as a marathon strategy is great for elite runners, but is it a good strategy for the non-elite runner? The short answer is astoundingly yes. We will now shift focus on speed variations in non-elite runners, those finishing a marathon between three hours and thirty minutes and beyond.

We commonly observe non-elite runners starting the marathon fast, but they go fast for too long. These runners did not know how to "let go" of this fast start before the fifth kilometer and did not run by varying their speed. Studying the times each kilometer in a marathon of non-elite runners (3 hours and 30 minutes – 4 hours), shows a linear downward trend that intersects the average time around the half marathon point. Next, there is an attempt to "rebound and hold" over the next 5 – 10 km. In the last 10 km before the final "sprint" (the call of the finish line!), they are often running much slower than they started. These runners started quickly, allowing them to get ahead while their muscles were fresh, but by not slowing down, they fatigued and cracked near the finish.

Remember that non-elite runners have a distribution of their speeds to the left. This distribution means that they spend more time and distance above their average speeds and then collapse after trying in vain to maintain this constant overestimated speed. Even an elite runner like Haile Gebrselassie has been known to do this as we can see in Figure 11. He attempted the world record using the strategy of maintaining a speed to the point of fatigue, and the result is a "failed" race.

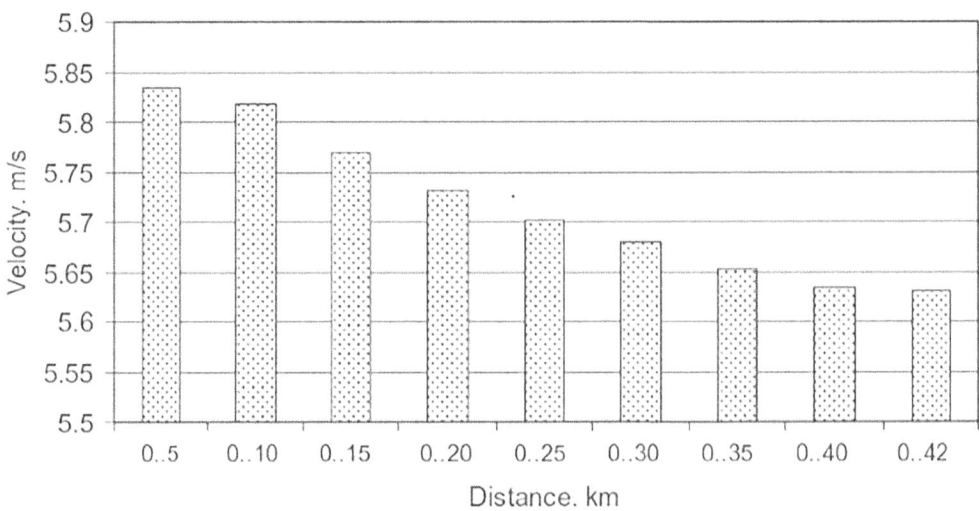

Figure 11. Cumulative time, pace, and velocity at the 2008 Dubai Marathon. Up to the 15th km, Haile Gebrselassie and his pacers were on track for a new world record under 2 hours and 2 minutes but ultimately fell short (Erdmann and Lipinska 2013).

SPEED FREQUENCY HISTOGRAMS

One of the several tools we use at BillaTraining.com is speed frequency histograms. The speed frequency histogram of your marathon quickly allows you to see the distribution of your speeds; it shows how much you have run above and below your recurring speed or the speed which is "typical" for you. Recall, that the mode in statistics, is your dominant speed or the value that is most represented in your marathon. Exceptionally good non-elite runners whose finishing times are usually within 2 hours and 18 minutes – 2 hours and 25 minutes, run a balanced race with their dominant speeds centered around their average pace. We usually see an equivalent distribution between the distance and the time spent above and below the average running speed. In Figure 12, this runner's mode is 5.02 meters per second (5:31 mile/min) and is used more than eight hundred times. Given that speed is recorded every second, this represents 800 seconds or more than 13 minutes. Even more, this runner has a similar second speed that is also used more than eight hundred times, which in total gives nearly 30 minutes run at more than 5 m/s. (5:21 min/mile).

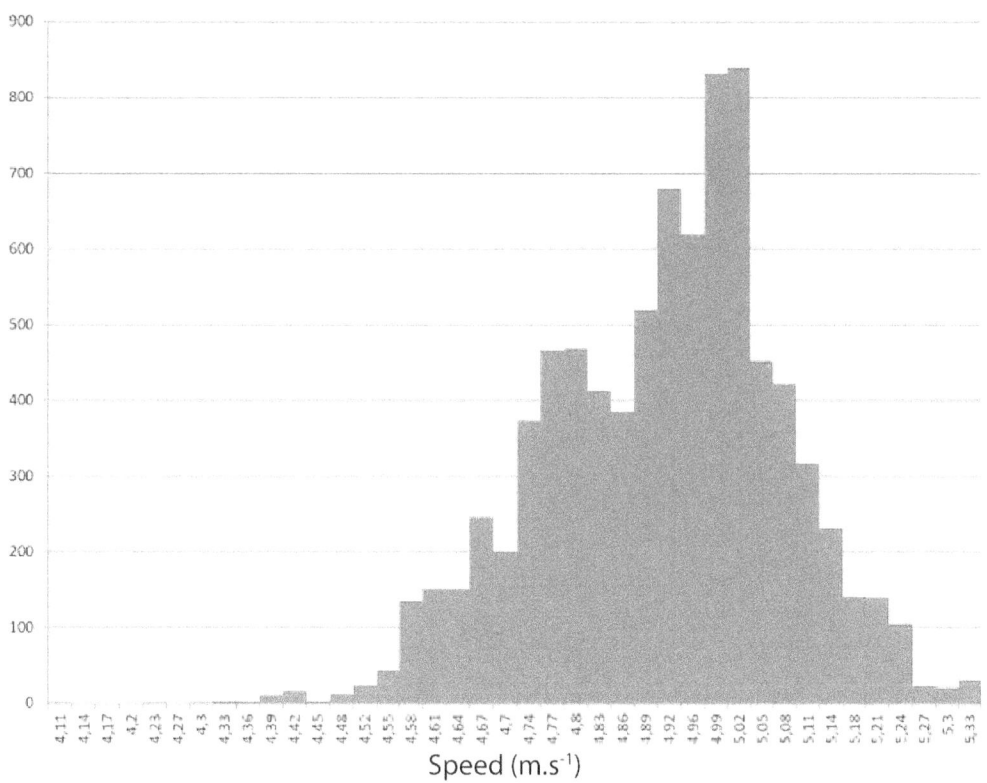

Figure 12. Histogram of a runner's speed frequencies during a marathon.

BOX PLOTS

In addition to the speed distribution histograms, we also have another simple tool: box plots. They allow us to visualize the distribution of the speeds. This allows a comparison of different runners or our own races. Notice in Figure 12, the large distributions of average speeds when we analyze the speed each second. In this group of runners whose performances range from 2:18 to 3:40, we find that the non-elite runners in this group spend more time running above than below, their average speed. This can be explained by the fact that they cannot run much above their average marathon pace because of a low-speed reserve. In addition, they fatigue and crack without the possibility of running above their average speed. On the contrary, the best runners have a superposition between their average speeds and their medians (a reminder: the median separates 50/50 the periods of time run at the top speed and below the average). Finally, exceptional runners like Haile Gebrselassie have a convex-type race (in the form of a bowl), allowing them to slow down and run below their average speed due to a fast start and the ability to accelerate in the last third of the race. For the elite runner, the winning strategy is one that allows you to set your PR without being out of competition for three months. A convex-type speed variation may be adequate for a high-level runner but a little risky for an average runner who has not mastered variable speed running. Adopting a progressive speed reduction strategy, starting from a speed higher than the average speed of the target time is the idea.

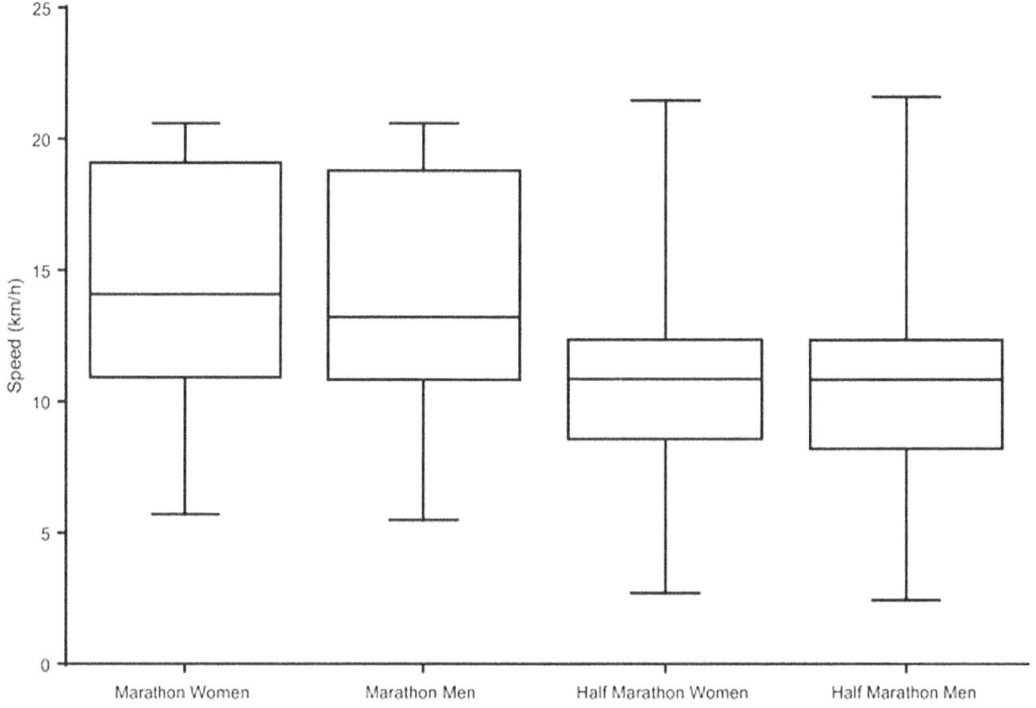

Figure 13. Boxplots to visualize the gap around the mean and extremes for a marathon and half-marathon runners (Knechtle 2016).

Around the "drop" in your speed, we will show you how to oscillate your pace while considering your physiological profile. Trusting our sensations is one of the harder things to do in running. The regulation of our speed is the result of a forward-looking plan and the readjustments of speed via biofeedback from physiological sensations (Billat 2018). The main benefit for analyzing your speed variation model is that it gives you confidence that the effect of varying the speed is the optimization of energy.

We are not implying that you need to track your times every meter of the marathon. Simply, we must free ourselves from the idea that a constant pace is the best way to progress and perform. **No researcher has found the constant physiological speed that allows both fatigue resistance and one to run as quickly as possible over a given distance**. Research models that determine marathon performance run at a constant speed on a treadmill, are dangerous. We are showing this in a research paper where we analyzed more than two-hundred marathons on Strava®. It is predictable that all runners finishing in 2 hours and 30 minutes or more, ran at near a constant speed until the 17th mile (two-thirds of the race) and then experienced fatigue (which must be managed). Therefore, a proper race strategy must include a speed reduction plan for every 10-km (6 miles). Like anything in life, this skill must be practiced and mastered by learning the relationship between gait, physiologic sensations, and expectations.

DISSECTING YOUR MARATHON

Now, for the more curious among you, we will describe how to quantify a marathon performance beyond just a graph, as we did for Haile Gebrselassie. It is complex and something we do in the research lab. This is a challenge for the amateur marathoner due to the lack of precise speed measurements during a marathon. Quantifying the asymmetry of the breakdown of your marathon speeds above and below your average running speed is essential. The main interest in quantifying the marathon performance is to run less distance above your average speed and run in short waves at a pace higher than your average speeds. More precisely, it is necessary to run more distance below the average, but not too far below your average. The goal is to run about 2 km/h (1.24 mph) below your average; picture running in small oscillations (waves) whose height is lower than 2 km/h. With practice, you should be able to avoid fatigue and muscle acidosis. We notice (Figure 14) from the tenth segment of the marathon, a decrease in speed as the distance increases. The point here is that the trend is significant early in the race after the fourth km.

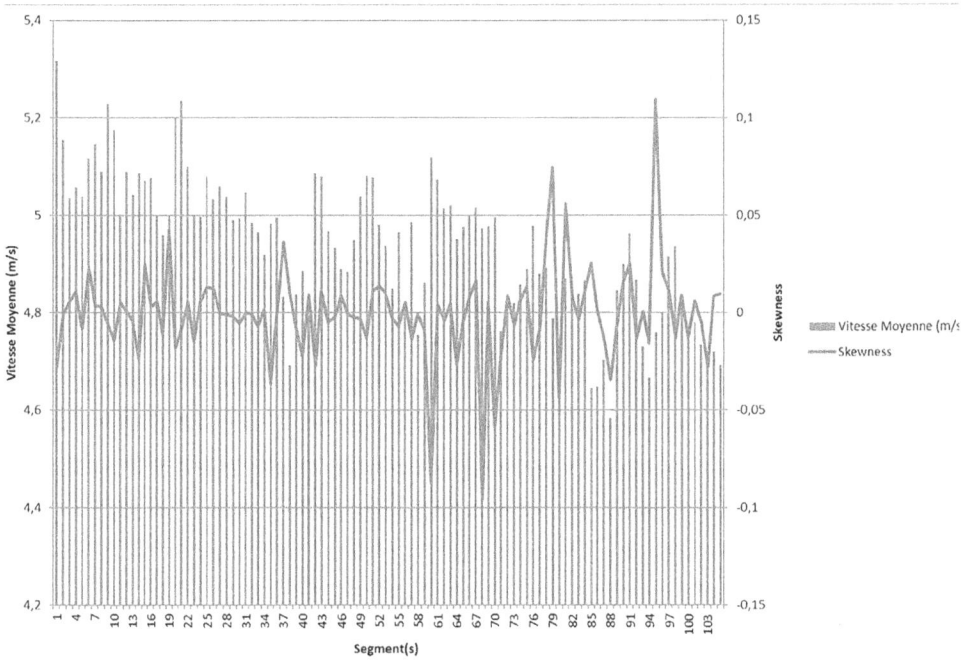

Figure 14. Evolution of a runner's (blue) race speed distribution as a function of the distance (400-meter range) during a marathon. The red curve is the asymmetry coefficient (skewness) of the speed distribution at 400-m intervals. The asymmetry to the left of the average (and therefore lower) speed of the segment (value of the negative asymmetry) is very marked in the sixtieth segment of 400-m. The runner tries to catch up with the seventy-sixth segment (32nd km) by a positive asymmetry i.e. an above-average speed distribution and an acceleration at the end of the race.

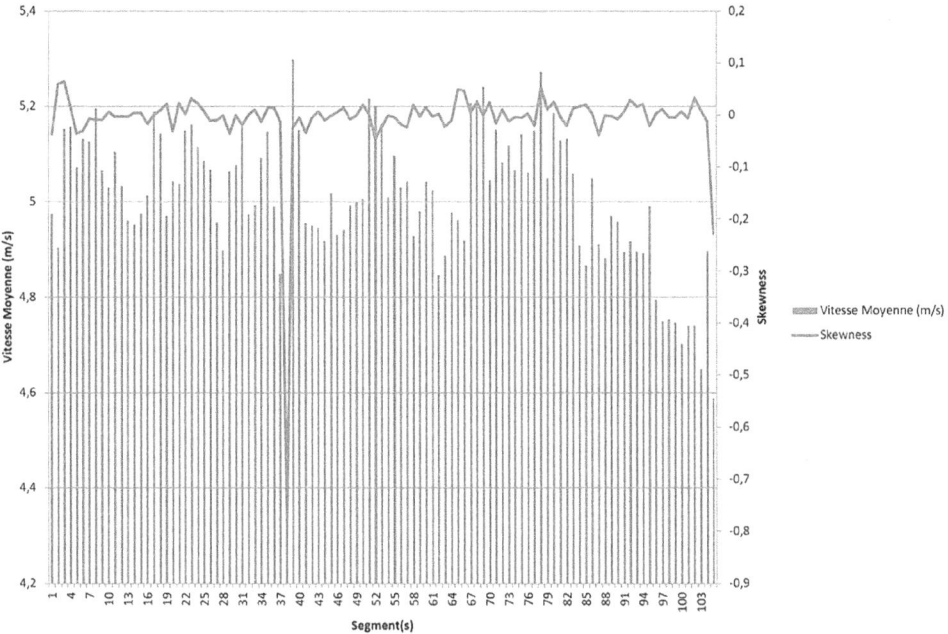

Figure 15. Speed signature of a runner who manages to maintain overall high speed by oscillations that partially compensate for a fall in trend speed.

Overall, after reviewing the distribution of the running speeds in Figure 15 compared to the average speed for each 400-m segment, we can work out the asymmetry coefficient, the mean, the median, and the mode as well as the downward trend in speed over the entire race. The most frequent speed (the mode) is both greater than the median speed and higher than the average speed of the calculated marathon dividing the distance of the runner by the final time (distance/running time 8578 seconds or 2 hours and 22 minutes). This means that the race has a tendency of loss of speed and that the asymmetry coefficient is low (close to 0), and an average speed is close to the median speed. The speed mode, which is the most frequent speed of this runner, is above the average and median speeds which means that the runner often returns to this higher speed thanks to oscillations around this trend of linear decline (Figure 15). We note, in Figure 14, a less pronounced downward trend (because of this concavity) which shows a start that is too slow that the runner attempted to compensate for via an increase in speed at the halfway point, which was not favorable if we look at the end of race. After this complex mathematical analysis, and before addressing the underlying physiological and psychological factors, let's go back to the basics and recall the five golden rules to succeed in your marathon:

FIVE GOLDEN RULES FOR MARATHON SUCCESS

The Start

Do not resist the euphoria of the start. Everything you have worked for is about the start. Take it all in and go with a fast start even if it seems too much for 1 or 2 km. This allows you to take advantage of your fresh legs and launching your aerobic engine faster.

Get into Your zone

Do not be afraid to watch your times and start getting into your mindset using music or however you achieve this. Don't let yourself be distracted by looking for your friends, a colleague in the race, or the people on the side. Do not listen to encouragements. Automatically, you will find yourself letting go if you start fast enough. It will be even more beneficial since you will be gone quickly, and you will do it from the first kilometer.

Find Your Comfort Zone and Rhythm

Once you have found your rhythm, try to run maintaining small oscillations using your sensations. Try to vary the stride which will decrease the stress on the muscles. This way you will have the time to regenerate your creatine phosphate (your premium gas!) and to recycle lactate to pyruvate and use it like glucose.

Use the Hydration Stations

Strategically use hydration stations. It is an essential stage of your race that you must not miss. The advice is to rinse your mouth or drink a sip of water and pour the rest on your head. Eat just a little to make your brain happy, perhaps a bar or if in France, an almond paté. For runs greater than 3 hours and 30 minutes, use crackers and cheese or rice cakes.

Do Not Worry About the Miles or Kilometers You Have Run

Do not worry about the distance already run, nor about what's left to run. Run in the moment! The information that is useful for the prediction of the future is entirely contained in the present. Nothing is dependent on the past. What counts for the speed variation model is not how you reached the twenty-first kilometer, but how you are now. For example, imagine that you are at the half-marathon point, which is symbolic of the philosophy of life; we can determine ourselves in the present state of our motivation. Our Cartesian education prevents us from being connected to ourselves, from having the fearlessness and self-confidence that is often called "small grain of madness" by reasonable people!

Let's be crazy and dream of the world record!

CHAPTER THREE SUMMARY

CONCEPT: The non-elite runners in this group spend more time running above, than below, their average speed. This can be explained by the fact that they cannot run much above their average marathon pace because of a low speed reserve. In addition, they fatigue and crack without the possibility of running above their average speed. On the contrary, the best runners have a superposition between their average speeds and their medians (a reminder: the median separates 50/50 the periods of time run at the top speed and below the average). Finally, exceptional runners such as Haile Gebrselassie have a convex type race (in the form of a bowl) allowing them to slow down and run below their average speed due to a great initial advance and the ability to accelerate in the last third of the race.

APPLICATION: A good strategy for success in a world record marathon is a U-shaped race pattern. It can be the difference between a successful elite runner setting a world record or PB, versus that of a failed race. You might be thinking that speed variation as a marathon strategy is great for elite runners, but is it a good strategy for the non-elite runner? The short answer is astoundingly yes. We will now shift focus on speed variations in non-elite runners, that is, those that can finish a marathon between three hours and thirty minutes and beyond. Around the "drop" in your speed, we will show you how to oscillate your pace while considering your physiological profile. One of the harder things to do in running is that we must trust our sensations. The regulation of our speed is the result of a forward-looking plan and the permanent readjustments of speed via biofeedback from physiological parameters (Billat 2018). The main benefit for analyzing your speed variation model is that it gives you confidence that the result of varying the speed is the optimization of energy.

CHAPTER 4

BREAKING THE 2-HOUR MARATHON AND SPEED VARIATION

In 2017, Nike launched a highly publicized attempt to break the 2-hour marathon on the Circuit of Monza (Italy), Eliud Kipchoge came within 25 seconds of running a sub-2-hour marathon. The attempt in Monza was built on the belief that constant speed is the best way of running. This idea is perpetuated by marathon organizers who offer pace group leaders to help the runners maintain a target speed. A sub-2-hour marathon requires a strict pace of 2 minutes and 50 seconds per kilometer (4:33 min/mile). The runners used over thirty pacers (known in the running world as rabbits) rotated in formation every two km. Because the three athletes in the Nike challenge ran with a roster of interchangeable pacers, this violates IAAF regulations and Kipchoge's time was not official. However, he does hold the current world marathon record of 2:01:39 (Berlin 2018).

In 2019, INEOS supported the 2-hour attempt, and Kipchoge achieved the historic milestone in Vienna, Austria, with a time of 1 hour 59 minutes and 40 seconds. However, his result is not recognized as a world record, but rather an exhibition marathon. Nevertheless, he is the first person in history to run a marathon in less than two hours. Kipchoge, age thirty-four, achieved a sports milestone granted almost mythical status in the running world, just as when Sir Roger Bannister broke the 4-minute mile. The fact that someone ran a sub-2-hour marathon will be a mental boost to the running world because we now know that it can be done, and others will undoubtedly follow.

Breaking the sub-2-hour marathon was achieved in a "fabricated" manner, certainly not how we would go about it, but it did accomplish its goals. The Nike Breaking2 and INEOS projects were organized to break the 2-hour barrier for the marathon. Several issues exist with this sub-2-hour marathon effort. In our opinion, the performance by Kipchoge was a materialistic, anti-physiologic effort as it applies to marathon running. Kipchoge — who wore a white singlet, white sneakers, carbon-fiber-plated Nike prototype shoes (only recently released to the public) — had immense support. He ran behind an electric timing car driving 4:34 per mile with rotating pacesetters (thirty-five on the course, six on reserve), which included some of the best distance runners in the world, including the former world and Olympic gold medalists Bernard Lagat and Matthew Centrowitz. This marathon was anti-physiological because none of the runners ran according to their sensations. Neither Kipchoge nor his pacers were allowed to pace themselves, and they were always constrained by the pace car. It would have been much better if Kipchoge could have paced himself and the car used as a wind block. The runners had no opportunity to change or vary speeds according to their physiology and experience. The possibility of running a sub-2-hour marathon in a real race, using the runner's sensations, varying the pace, and not a constant pace, is real. Nevertheless, Kipchoge, the Olympic marathon champion (Rio 2016), was able to cut 1 minute and 14 seconds into his world record (2 hours 1 minute 39 seconds, Berlin 2018) and 2 minutes and 32 seconds into the previous world record held by his compatriot Dennis Kimetto (2 hours 2 minutes 57 seconds, Berlin 2014).

In the 2017 attempt, the team of three elite runners was Eluid Kipchoge (Kenya), Zersenay Tadese (Eritrea), and Lelisa Desisa (Ethiopia). Monza was chosen as a venue because of its near sea-level altitude, mild weather conditions, and short lap length. Nike also brought in thirty of the world's best runners to serve as pacers, with the likes of Sam Chelanga, Chris Derrick, Bernard Lagat, and Andrew Bumbalough. Unlike in a real marathon, the pacemaker vehicles and the pacers were positioned in a V-shape, providing a wind block for the three runners. A green laser beam projecting from the pace car always indicated where the runners needed to be. The event began in light rain at 5:45 am, and the temperature was about 54 degrees F (12 degrees C). A constant pace of 4:34.50 per mile or 2:50 per kilometer is required to break the 2-hour barrier. The runners started on pace, but both Desisa and Tadese fell off the pace at kilometers 16 and 20, respectively. Kipchoge remained on pace until the thirtieth km, where he was off by only 1 second. Ultimately, Kipchoge came up 25 seconds short of running under 2 hours. This is a shame because Kipchoge, Tadese, and Desisa, had this record in their legs. But they needed to rethink their approach to the race and consider that holding a constant speed is not ideal. There are many factors at play, but the energy cost and the increase in body temperature change the perception of the race's difficulty at constant or non-varying speeds.

THE POSSIBILITY OF A SUB-2-HOUR MARATHON USING A VARIABLE PACE STRATEGY

These three runners were tested and validated on an energy strategy based on the calculation of VO2 max. VO2 max is based on thirty-year-old thinking and does not tell us if a runner can finish at a specific time. VO2 max corresponds to the speeds producing 3 – 4 mmol/L of lactate on an incremental VAMEVAL treadmill test. VAMEVAL means VAM EVAL or evaluation of VAM. The term VAM is confusing and is an Italian abbreviation for *velocita ascensionale media*, which translates into the mean ascent velocity. The VAMEVAL test is a running exercise used to calculate the speed at VO2 max, which will be covered later.

We believe that it is no longer necessary to search systematically for the runner who will be able to beat the marathon world record based on VO2 max or energy cost (Physiology and Methodology of Training, Billat 2017). VO2 max is based on the paradigm of constant velocity from the equation of Pietro di Prampero:

$$V \text{ marathon (m/min)} = F \times VO2 \text{ max}/CE$$

where V marathon is the speed in meters per minute, VO2 max in ml/min/kg (from 40 to 88 ml/min/kg), and F is the fraction of VO2 max (aerobic power factor) used during the marathon (60 to 80 percent depending on the endurance of the runner), and energy cost (CE) of the race in milliliters of oxygen consumed per meter and per kilometer (from 0.180 to 0.210 ml/kg per meter from most to least economic).

By taking the best values recorded in the world-class runners, this gives a V marathon or speed (m/min) = (0.8 × 88) / 0.180 = 391 m/min or 23 km/h, or 1 hour and 48 minutes in the marathon. The 2-hour marathon record can indeed be broken in a real race.

It is essential to realize that this thirty-year-old thinking of using VO2 max to establish records is false. It is false because the estimation of the fractional utilization of VO2 max (F) at 80 percent (0.8) is derived from a lactate production of 3 mmol/L. A more in-depth look into estimating the arbitrary lactate value of 3 mmol/L shows that it is flawed. These values are based upon incremental treadmill tests (VALMEVAL) for which the re-oxidation of lactate cannot be reused. It is well known that humans can achieve balanced lactate levels of 8 mmol/L while running at variable speeds based on the feelings of the runner (Figure 16).

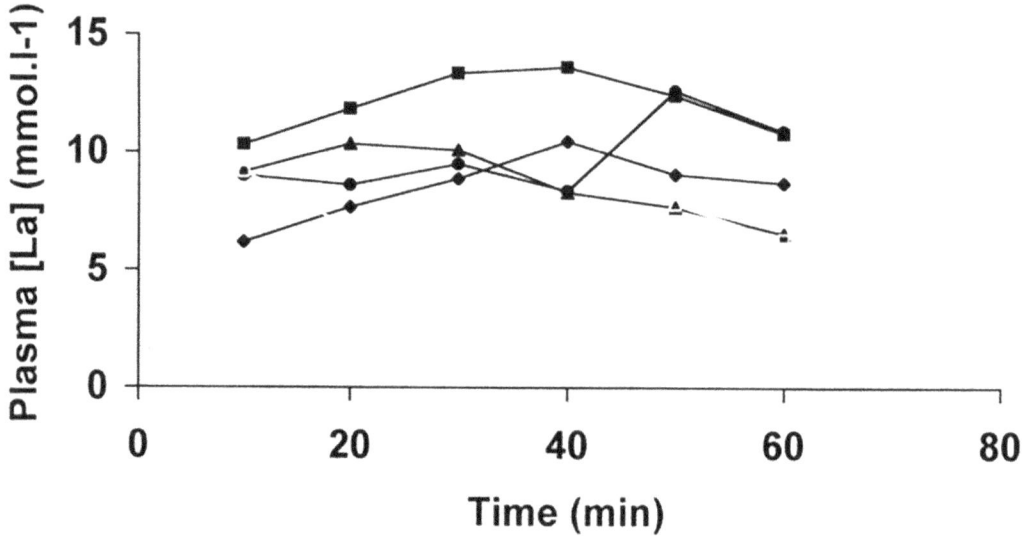

Figure 16. Individual values of blood lactate concentration for four subjects with the highest averages at 10 – 50 minutes. The maximum stable state of lactate as a function of time can exist well above four mmol/L, especially when variable speeds are used (Myburgh 2001).

Running at constant speed requires exceptional qualities that are difficult to obtain in the same runner. The high VO2 max values are often associated with higher oxygen costs, which is precisely what allows runners to reach a high VO2 max. Candidates for the sub-2-hour marathon record possessed the physiological and performance criteria per the equations above. They did not require running at a constant speed (behind a car, with alternating pacers, and a car emitting a laser beam).

The best performances of Eliud Kipchoge on different distances are summarized below.

- 10,000-m at 26 minutes and 49 seconds
- 1500-m in 3 minutes and 33 seconds
- 3000-m in 7 minutes and 26 seconds

These performances mean that Eliud Kipchoge has a large physiologic reserve of power, which allows him to vary his speed during a long race such as the marathon.

Summary of the Breaking2 project:

Presentation of the three candidates for the 2017 Breaking2 sub-2-hour marathon by Nike

- ELIUD KIPCHOGE (KENYA): thirty-five years old on the day of the race/final time: 2 hours and 25 seconds. Eliud is an Olympic marathon champion with eleven wins in twelve races, and he is one of the best athletes in his discipline. His world record time of 2 hours 1 minute and 39 seconds (Berlin 2018), is the fastest time in official marathon history. Eluid Kipchoge's best chronometric performances over different distances:

Distance	Time	Date	Place
1500 m	3 min 33s	May 2004	Hengelo
3000 m	7 min 27 s	May 2011	Doha
5000 m	12 min 46 s	July 2004	Rome
10000 m	26 min 42 s	May 2007	Hengelo
10 km	28 min 11 s	September 2009	Utrecht
Half Marathon	59 min 25 s	September 2012	Lille
Marathon	2 h 1 min 39 s	September 2018	Berlin

- ZERSENAY TADESE (ERITREA): thirty-four years old on race day/final time: 2 hours 6 minutes and 51 seconds. Zersenay has won four Olympic medals and five World Half Marathon Championships. He holds the current record for the men's half marathon with a time of fifty-eight minutes and 23 seconds. Running was not the first choice of Zersenay. As a teenager, he wanted to be a professional cyclist before being spotted by track and field recruiters. Chronometric performances of Zersenay Tadese (he does not have an official reference for the marathon):

Distance	Time	Date	Place
3000 m	7 min 39 s	May 2005	Doha
5000 m	12 min 59 s	July 2006	Rome
10000 m	26 min 37 s	Aug 2006	Brussels

- LELISA DESISA (ETHIOPIA): twenty-seven years old on the day of the race/final time: 2 hours 14 minutes and 10 seconds. Lelisa is the youngest of the group, and yet, during the Dubai Marathon in 2013, he ran one of the fastest marathon times in history as a rookie with 2 hours 4 minutes and 45 seconds. A two-time winner of the Boston Marathon (2013 and 2015), and he posted a PB of fifty-nine minutes and 30 seconds in the half marathon. Lelisa Desisa's best chronometric performances over different distances:

Distance	Time	Date	Place
5000 m	13 min 22 s	June 2012	Rome
10000 m	27 min 18 s	June 2012	Liege
Half Marathon	59 min 30 s	Nov 2011	New Delhi
Marathon	2 h 4 min 45 s	Jan 2013	Dubai

Notice that the two best runners were the oldest (thirty-five and thirty-four years old). Zersenay Tadese has no experience in the marathon. Nevertheless, he held the world record for the half-marathon. Lelisa Desisa, a two-time Boston Marathon champion, cracked at the halfway point of the record attempt. It is important to note that the Boston marathon course is uneven and involves varying lengths of stride and speed (therefore race power), which will become apparent in a later chapter. Monza is flat and was strictly run at constant speed! At BillaTraining.com, we are betting that an attempt at a real sub-2-hour marathon will come from a runner with variable speeds based on times according to his physiology. All these runners have large reserves of power, speed, and the capability to run a marathon in under two hours, they just need to be allowed to do so.

We have created a marathon model using speed distributions that would allow a runner to achieve a sub-2-hour marathon without having extraordinary VO2 max values. For example, by taking a runner with a VO2 max of 80 ml/min/kg and a 10-km time less than 26 minutes and 57 seconds, we can see that this corresponds to the profile of the runners in the Breaking2 project at Monza in 2017. It is noteworthy that one-hundred runners in the world have already run this 10-km time, and to date, we have over six hundred potential candidates. For a runner with a 10-km time of 27 minutes, the maximum speed of our marathon will only be equal to 102 percent of the average speed over 10-km (speed held over 3 minutes at the beginning of the race). Also, it will be well below the top speed of the 10-km. We must go beyond the notions of speed target calculations from the average times over 10-km and the half marathon. We dare to say that the speed variations in training methods are valuable for the marathon and other races. That's why a good season of cross-country running and cross-country skiing over four to six weeks in December or January, for example, are excellent winter preparation methods for the Boston Marathon in April.

Setpoint	Top speed of the zone (km/h)	Lower speed of the zone (km/h)
Sprint	29	25
Very hard	24	22
Hard	21	19
Average	18	16

Table 1. Zone profile of perceived speed from easy to sprint required to pass the 2-hour barrier to the marathon. A VO2 max of "only" 80.5 ml/kg/min is required to break the world record with a variable speed strategy, unlike the constant speed race at Monza for the Breaking2 project.

Looking at the runners' profiles who attempted to break the 2-hour marathon in 2017, it is clear that we have the ingredients to break the world marathon record with a not-so-extraordinary speed profile (Table 1). If we observe the speed distributions, mainly the average speed, we can preconceive this simulation of a sub-2-hour marathon, with a small increase in the frequency of higher speeds in the three-fourths of the upper distribution (3rd quartile). This small period of higher speeds (in relation to the average) corresponds to a rapid start, emphasizing the strategy of advancing the speed reserve in a fresh state with the ability to give it everything you have in the last 30 minutes (ten 3-minute intervals).

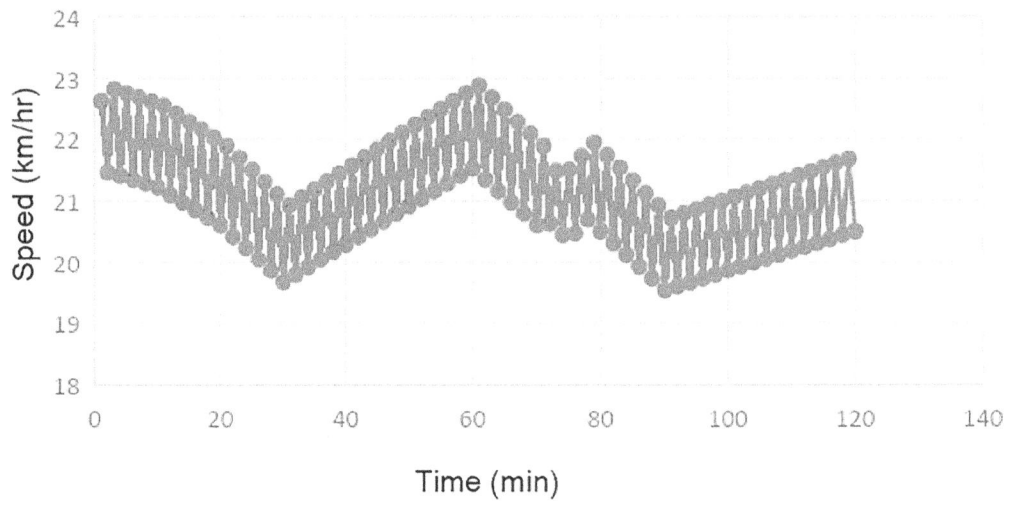

Figure 17. Speed signature (zone) to set the world record in less than 2 hours. With references in VO2 max and chronometric over 10 km, there are more than one hundred runners fall within these criteria.

With a fast start, "letting go" early, and speed oscillations corresponding to what a runner does naturally when he settles into an average pace, a runner can produce a faster finish in the last 10 minutes of the race. The three runners of the Breaking2 project would have the ability to follow this race plan since the margin of safety is large according to their 10-km and half-marathon records.

The key to success in the marathon is a large physiologic power reserve. Earlier in the book, we highlighted that what made the difference between marathoners who run less than 2 hours and 11 minutes compared to those between 2 hours and 11 minutes and 2 hours and 16 minutes **was surprisingly the best speed over 1000-m**. The notion that power is closely linked to running speed is often overlooked. Power (watts or joules/s) is directly related to the economy of running, which is the consumption of oxygen (in ml O2/kg/min). But there is an energy equivalent between the oxygen consumed and the mechanical work produced. For each milliliter of oxygen consumed, 20.9 J of mechanical energy are created from one gram of glucose and a little less from fat, which requires more oxygen to burn. All of this means that this volume of oxygen consumed per minute, the infamous VO2 max is comparable to power.

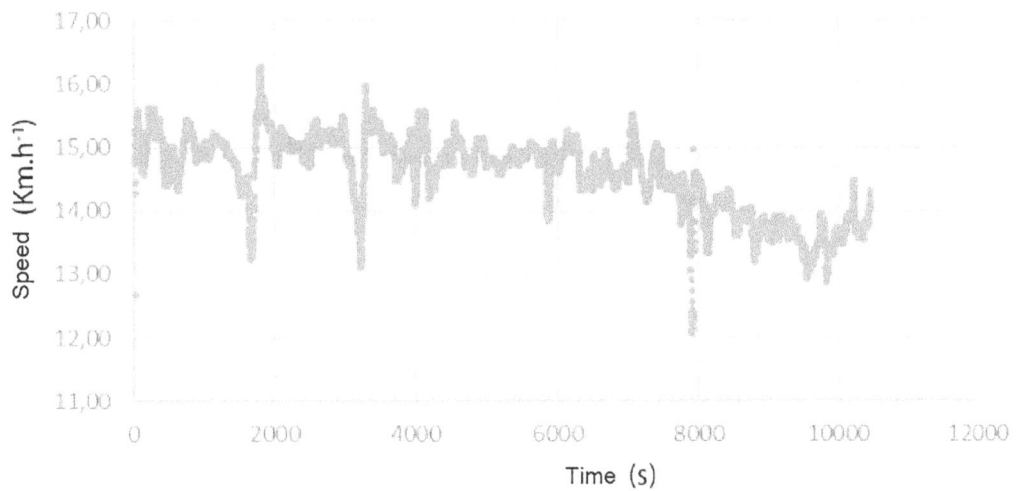

Figure 18. Racing strategy (speed) set up by a runner during a marathon. This runner suffered in his race. Indeed, he tried, at all costs, to maintain a constant speed estimated from 75 percent of his MAS.

How to Shave 10 Minutes off Your Marathon Time

A piece of advice for the marathon runner who currently runs a marathon in about 3 hours, and wants to improve their time by 10 minutes, is the necessity to race more intelligently. It is possible to compensate for the lack of physical qualities with age by racing with "intelligence." The first step is to review the runner's race pattern. Then by practicing the methods in this book and learn to start fast for 1–2 km. Next, learn to decrease the

> pace below their average speed and run by oscillating the speed by 1 – 2 km/hr always guided by his/her sensations. This will allow the runner to spend more time below his/her average speed, giving them the energy to finish strong. In contrast to the marathon runner in Figure 18, he ruined his efforts by a drastic fall in his race speed after the thirtieth kilometer, which will show that he spent more time above his final average speed! It may be counter-intuitive, but to succeed in your marathon, you must listen to your wise laziness!

CHAPTER FOUR SUMMARY

CONCEPT: Thanks to a fast start, an early "letting go," and speed oscillations that correspond to what the runner does naturally when he settles into an "average" feeling, he can produce a faster finish in the last 10 minutes of the race. The three runners of the Breaking2 project can follow this race plan since the margin of safety, as seen in their 10-km and half-marathon records, is large for the three runners. The key to success in the marathon is having a large physiologic power reserve. Earlier in the book, we highlighted that what made the difference between marathoners who run less than 2 hours and 11 minutes compared to those between 2 hours and 11 minutes and 2 hours and 16 minutes **was surprisingly the best speed just 1000 m**. The notion that power is directly linked to running speed is often overlooked.

APPLICATION: A piece of advice for a marathon runner who currently runs a marathon in about 3 hours, and wants to improve their time by 10 minutes, is the necessity to race more intelligently. It is possible to compensate for the lack of physical qualities with age by using better "intelligence" during the race. The first step is to review the runner's race pattern. By practicing the methods in this book and learning to start fast for 1 to 2 km, then decreasing the pace below their average speed and oscillating the speed by 1-2 km/hr always guided by his/her sensations. The runner will be able to spend more time below his/her average speed, and then have the energy to finish strong.

CHAPTER 5
THE PHYSIOLOGICAL FOUNDATIONS OF CLASSICAL ENDURANCE TRAINING

MAS AND VO2 MAX AND MAXIMAL LACTATE STABLE STATE (MLSS) THRESHOLDS IN ENDURANCE

THE MINDSET OF ENDURANCE TRAINING in the 1980s (which still governs us today) was built on an exercise model of constant speed and, even worse, at incremental speeds validated on a treadmill. One goal of this chapter is to explain the endless streams of misinformation found on "specialized" running websites. Original training methods (or the so-called classical method) were developed in exercise physiology laboratories using treadmills at constant or incremental speeds with VAMEVAL protocols. Recall that the VAMEVAL protocol is an Italian acronym for "Velocidad Aerobie Maximale EVALuation." Whenever you see the word VAMEVAL, you know that it is an incremental treadmill test. We will see that these theories of the metabolic pathways and force-velocity power are based on monotonous, robotic training cycles.

Moreover, it was these theories that recommended high mileage training volumes such as LSD training. These training methods ultimately lead to a "cul-de-sac" or dead-end, eventually resulting in chronic injuries, overtraining, and a decreased desire to run. The training consisted primarily of short and long intervals (200 – 400-m and 800 – 2000-m) and tempo training at race-specific speeds or at the anaerobic threshold to improve the MAS and VO2 max. Remember, that muscular power is the first limiting factor of oxygen consumption. Our lab has worked hard at developing alternative physiological parameters such as VO2 max and MAS.

TRADITIONAL HIGH MILEAGE RUNNING IS RISKY

To run a marathon, many coaches build a program around a foundation of easy-to-medium paced running with an emphasis on building up the total weekly mileage. Historically, this is known as the long, slow, distance method, or LSD for short. The principle of LSD running is that it is aerobic and slow, and therefore trains explicitly those muscle fibers that have more mitochondria, and as a result, use a lot of oxygen. Building up these systems is essential to increase metabolic flexibility and decrease the likelihood of bonking after the twentieth mile. LSD-type training's physiologic benefits are increased fat burning, blood capillary density, mitochondrial density, tendon and ligament strength, improved bone density, and, most of all, improved oxygen utilization. A primary advantage of LSD-type programs is that it increases the body's ability to burn fat. Ironically, many runners build their fat burning capacity yet subsist on high carbohydrate gels. Traditional exercise physiologists prescribed the LSD model of endurance training to prepare the body for speed work and high-level racing with the rational of the more you run, the better. Building up weekly mileage is essential in any long-distance event, especially the marathon. But it should be done by optimizing your natural sensations to running. It is unnecessary to run hundreds of miles per week, and some research suggests that anything over 75 miles per week is not worth the risk. Most LSD-type programs are about 60 miles or more per week for amateurs, and many elite marathoners take this advice to extremes and run 100 – 150 miles per week and sometimes more. It is undoubtedly true that LSD-type training can produce results, but at what cost? Attaining these results are great if you avoid injury or chronic pains. Quality must be mixed with quantity to produce maximum results.

High mileage running leads to injuries in 90 percent of marathon runners (calves, shin splints, and arch injuries) based on quality research. One of our goals at BillaTraining.com is to ensure you can reach a higher level of fitness while avoiding injuries. LSD training leads to a decrease in mobility, range of motion, decrease in strength, muscular imbalances, and postural weakness. A significant number of runners get stress fractures caused by an excessive training load. Even more, chronic training leads to adverse effects on the body, such as decreased cortisol, hormones like testosterone, and taxing the immune system.

Another caveat of LSD running is that if you, by chance, avoid injury, you will be predominantly good at running slow speeds. More importantly, you will lack the ability to accelerate and recover. Most runners who follow traditional high mileage training programs will peak at about 20 miles in a marathon. This is the reason why those last 6.2 miles are often so agonizing for many runners. Adapting your body to start fast while your muscles are fresh, and then letting go of the pace and running under your average, will allow you to finish those last miles much easier. It took thirty years of research to show that a minimalistic training program, decreasing mileage, adding higher intensities, increasing strength, and optimizing running economy is the better way forward. The lower rate of injuries is one of the main benefits. Weight training and activities such as jump rope improve tendons' and ligaments' strength and bone density. Of all the physiologic benefits that LSD-type training provides, a minimalistic, acceleration-based training program using your sensations does better.

Dr. Billat's research shows that slow-to-moderate constant paced running does not improve running economy, lactate threshold and utilization, and injury prevention compared to acceleration-based workouts. Higher intensity training optimizes the neuro-muscular patterns, which improves the recruitment muscle fibers in the legs, boosting power, coordination, and speed; it even shows improvements in fatigue resistance and increased fat burning, resulting in less bonking at the twentieth mile. Research involving the central governor theory shows that improving these neuro-muscular connections may be the key to reaching a higher level of performance.

Adopting a minimalistic training regimen is a serious business. Think about it, even Olympic athletes, who have more resources than most marathon runners, become injured. Modern society has lost the connection between health and injury. Being able to listen to your body will achieve running freely without injury. Some coaches believe that weight training slows you down, increases body weight, and takes training time away. But studies are showing the opposite effects. Explosive exercises are resulting in significant gains in fatigue resistance, running economy, and faster run times.

> ### What is Fitness?
>
> There is no great definition of fitness. We can say that Kipchoge is among the fittest athletes in the world or that Kobe Bryant was among the fittest athletes who ever played the sport of basketball. Finally, Cristiano Ronaldo plays football (soccer) with amazing strength, agility, balance, and power; even more, he is rarely injured over the course of seventy games per year. It is important to discuss what is fitness and who is fit. Marathon running is a great sport, but we must realize that the fitness derived from marathon running is from increases aerobic and muscular efficiency. Fitness, in the real sense, is a continuum of general physical skills.
>
> The general physical skills that contribute to marathon running are cardiovascular endurance, stamina, strength, power, speed, coordination, flexibility, balance, and accuracy. You are as fit as you are competent in each of these skills. These skills come about through training and cardiorespiratory endurance, while others come about through practice, such as coordination. These skills are enhanced by developing the major metabolic pathways: phosphate, glycolytic, and oxidative pathways. Exercises such as the deadlift and squat elicit profound neuroendocrine responses. It is true that marathon runner's advance their fitness under a narrow bandwidth of functional capacity. Learning to do pull-ups and squats will make you a better runner. Having a meaningful understanding of what fitness is and how it affects us in the long term is useful. A particularly good book on this subject is *CrossFit Endurance*, written by Brian Mackenzie.

Developing our training programs was by no means easy, as our methods go against the grain of many established models. Training based on the different zones while varying the speed is not easy to understand or study. Measuring the characteristic changes involved with zones of variation of speeds was only possible by taking the laboratory outside. Tools such as portable gas analyzers, cardiac monitoring, and GPS-based measurements made it possible to develop and verify our training protocols. To clarify the notions of classic training preached in magazines, the Internet, and in running clubs, we will give you precise and straightforward explanations of these physiological concepts that have underpinned the classic training methods.

MAS AND VO2 MAX – WHAT THEY MEAN

Maximal Aerobic Speed (MAS)

Maximal aerobic speed or MAS is a term that you will see throughout this book, and it is an important part of developing your marathon training program. MAS is simply the lowest running speed at which maximum oxygen uptake (VO2 max) occurs. It is typically referred to as the velocity at VO2 max and written as MAS or vVO2 max. Said in another way, MAS is the slowest speed that elicits VO2 max. For example, a runner can reach their MAS and continue to run even faster, even though he/she has attained VO2 max. Physiologists and coaches use many tests to find a runners' MAS and prescribe appropriate training programs. It is important to clarify MAS and vVO2 max; they mean exactly the same thing and are used throughout the book. For clarity, we will try to use MAS as much as possible.

Another concept is the anaerobic velocity reserve. It is simply the difference between MAS and maximal sprint speed. For example:

An athlete has the following:

- MAS = 5.0 m/s
- Maximal Sprint Speed = 10.0 m/s
- Anerobic Velocity Reserve = 5.0 m/s

Before we dive into what MAS and VO2 max mean, it is important to highlight why these concepts are essential for you to understand during your marathon journey. VO2 max is a straightforward concept for those who have a science background. VO2 max has many names: maximal oxygen consumption, maximal oxygen uptake, and maximal aerobic capacity. VO2 max is simply the maximum rate of oxygen consumption measured during an incremental exercise of increasing intensity. VO2 max contains three abbreviations: V for volume, O2 for oxygen, and max for maximum. Maximal oxygen consumption reflects cardio-respiratory fitness and endurance capacity in exercise performance. VO2 max is vital in our everyday lives as it is an indicator of not only fitness but also human longevity. The American Heart Association published a statement recommending that VO2 max be regularly assessed and utilized as a vital sign, just like heart rate and temperature. Low VO2 max values are associated with early death, cancer, and all-cause mortality. Our bodies inhale oxygen and exhale carbon dioxide. Our cells do the same thing, and VO2 is a simple way to say that our cells take in oxygen and put out carbon dioxide. VO2 max is the point when this process hits a plateau.

THE DIFFERENCES BETWEEN MAS AND VO2 MAX.

Explaining VO2 max in the simplest of terms: VO2 max is simply the speed at which your body uses oxygen up to a maximal point. It refers to the maximum volume of oxygen that the body can use at maximum levels of intense aerobic exercise. It is usually reported as milliliters of oxygen used in 1 minute per kilogram of body weight, though sometimes you see liters of oxygen per minute with no adjustment for body weight. The former measurement is more useful in exercise and sports science since it allows for comparing athletes of various weights. It is a laboratory measurement performed on a treadmill or exercise bicycle where the athlete wears a mask connected to a machine that measures volume, oxygen, and carbon dioxide.

VO2 max is somewhat of a misnomer because it is the maximal oxygen consumption, but not the maximal speed achieved. It can exist over a range of values or speeds. Physiologists like to use the term MAS or vVO2 max to talk about the range in which VO2 max can exist for different speeds. MAS is simply the lowest speed at which maximal oxygen consumption or VO2 max occurs. In the scientific literature, it is also written as vVO2 max, which is the velocity at VO2 max. Since MAS or vVO2 max is the lowest speed at which a runner touches their VO2 max, there is a speed range at which MAS and VO2 max exist. It is also important to realize that MAS is only related to VO2 max, and it says nothing about running economy. To put this in perspective, a runner like Usain Bolt may reach their MAS at 21 mph (9.4 m/s), but their top sprint speed (also VO2 max) might be 27.8 mph (12.4 m/s). Since scientists like numbers in the metric system, we would say that Usain Bolt has an anaerobic speed reserve of 4 m/s.

WHY IS MAS USEFUL FOR RUNNING?

To better understand why MAS is useful for running, a little history helps. As MAS in relation to VO2 max was formalized in research, it was thought that it correlated with running performance because it considered running efficiency. Running at MAS was thought to be energy efficient since the speed at VO2 max is the ratio between a flow of energy and speed. Energy is estimated by the burning of glucose and fats while running, which is unique to everyone.

The idea of MAS came from the Cooper test, named after Kenneth Cooper MD, the Cooper Institute's founding doctor. Cooper was a military doctor who published the book *Aerobic Training* in 1968. In a sense, he was ahead of his time because he had connected the 12-minute distance and maximum oxygen consumption without any notion of MAS. The idea of MAS gained traction in the 1980s with Olympian Jack Daniels (silver medalist, Melbourne 1956). Daniels later became a professor of physiology, and he still coaches' runners and lives in Colorado. Jack Daniels invented the idea of MAS out of necessity. Measuring VO2 max in the 1980s was difficult due to the inconsistencies in results from one laboratory to another; this was due to poor calibration techniques and the lack of data automation. In 1998, Dr. Daniels published his famous book *The Daniels Running Formula* (Daniels 2014), offering interval training based on a runner's MAS, and everyone began using MAS in the running world.

THE IMPORTANCE OF TIME SPENT RUNNING AT MAS (T-LIM)

Once we have established a runner's MAS, measuring the maximum time spent at MAS is important. This means that we need to know the maximum amount of time a runner can hold the speed associated with his/her MAS. We accomplish this by having the runner warm-up and run at that speed correlating to his/her MAS until exhaustion. We call this value the time limit at MAS or T lim. In 1994, our laboratory proved that MAS was reproducible for an individual runner. We also showed that VO2 max alone did not predict performance. The 1994 article was one of the most internationally quoted in the field of exercise physiology between 1981 and 1996. With this information, we were better able to individualize interval training protocols when considering a runner's MAS and T lim. You do not need a large VO2 max to win races. Many marathon race winners have relatively low VO2 max scores. It means nothing to have a large VO2 max if the associated MAS was low due to an uneconomic stride.

RUNNING AND THE HYBRID ENGINE

We have already said that with an increase in running speed, the consumption of oxygen increases proportionally. In the simplest of terms, this means that to run faster, you must consume more oxygen per minute. Thus, oxygen consumption is a flow (a volume per unit of time) and is represented by the symbol V. In science journals, we use a point above the $\dot{V}$ which denotes a volume output by time. Keep in mind that this represents a volume of oxygen consumed per minute. Why should you consume more oxygen per minute to run faster? For humans, oxygen consumption (VO2) can be thought of like a complex hybrid engine. This hybrid engine produces locomotion following different energy paths. The main gas engine is thermal, burning glucose from glycogen and fatty acids from fat. Next, there are two different electric motors, which consist of a large and small battery. The large battery corresponds to the production and recycling of lactate, which is a result of glucose and fat metabolism. The small battery is the phospho-creatine shuttle in the mitochondria that produces locomotion for short periods of 1 to 3 seconds and does not require heat.

Our batteries are always recharging; we can recharge the small battery (phospho-creatine shuttle in the mitochondria) or using lactate in the big battery by eliminating waste (lactate recycling). The lactate produced, supplies energy to the heart to provide a minimum power (VO2 max) that will avoid complete unloading of the batteries. The small batteries can work without heat, akin to a complex hybrid engine, but only for 1 – 3 seconds since their discharge is akin to engaging the engine. The phospho-creatine shuttle helps you to accelerate quickly (from 0 to 20 km/h in 3 seconds, for example). Like a hybrid engine, we need to "burn" and oxidize more sugars (glucose molecules) per minute to provide the energy needed for muscle contraction. An excellent example of how vital these batteries are during exercise is when you are completely exhausted and cannot hold a pace. For example, this signifies that you have drained your batteries and are no longer adequately recharged.

THE ENERGY COST (CE) OF RUNNING

We know that in long-distance running, the largest volume of oxygen that can be consumed per minute per kilogram of body weight (VO2 max in ml/kg/min) is positively correlated with performance (Foster 1983). In other words, this is the maximum flow rate or maximum power of aerobic metabolism. However, for runners whose VO2 max values are comparable, the correlation between VO2 max and performance is weak. To better explain the differences between individual performances, we can compare the VO2 max and the CE. Thus, running performance can be improved either by increasing the fraction of the VO2 max sustained during the race, either by increasing the VO2 max, by reducing the CE of the race, or by any combination of these three parameters. The relation between VO2 max and energy cost (CE) is at the origins of the concept of speed at VO2 max. The determination of this speed is carried out either from physiological parameters (VO2 max and CE) or by measuring the highest speed reached during a progressive speed test to exhaustion. The speed at VO2 max makes it possible to establish a direct link between training performance and the determination of the speeds to be used during training. The velocity concept at VO2 max is a good illustration of the transfer of knowledge between research and its applications. In the literature, different protocols and abbreviations have been proposed to measure and identify velocity at VO2 max, which can be confusing (Hill and Rowell 1996).

CHAPTER 5 SUMMARY

CONCEPT: MAS, VO2 max, and MLSS Thresholds in Endurance composed the mindset of endurance training in the 1980s (which still governs us today). It was built on an exercise model of constant speed and, even worse, at incremental speeds validated on a treadmill. These theories of the metabolic pathways and force-velocity power are based on monotonous, robotic training cycles. Moreover, it was these theories that recommended high mileage training volumes such as LSD training. These training methods ultimately lead to a "cul-de-sac" or dead-end, eventually resulting in chronic injuries, overtraining, and a decreased desire to run.

APPLICATION: High mileage running leads to injuries in 90 percent of marathon runners (calves, shin splints, and arch injuries) based on well-done research. One of our goals at BillaTraining.com is to be sure you can attain the needed level of fitness, all the while avoiding injuries. LSD training leads to decrease mobility, range of motion, decreased strength, muscular imbalances, and postural weakness. A significant number of runners attain stress fractures caused by an excessive training load. Even more, chronic training leads to adverse effects on the body, such as a decreased cortisol reserve and other hormones like testosterone as well as taxing the immune system. Most runners who follow traditional mileage building marathon training programs will peak at about 20 miles. This is the reason why those last 6.2 miles are often so agonizing for many runners. Adapting your body to start fast while your muscles are fresh and then let go of the pace and run under your average will allow you to be able to run those last miles much easier.

CHAPTER 6

INCREASING YOUR SPEED RESERVE

IMAGINE RUNNING A MARATHON WITHOUT cracking, and with the pleasure of running it below your average speed for over half of the race. Running a marathon using speed variations is the key to finishing the event and enjoying the experience. Training using traditional lactate thresholds, the same plans, and the same MAS (10 and 25 percent above your average marathon speed), will never allow you to succeed in being able to vary your speed in a marathon. If you condemn yourself to always running at the same speed, it will induce the unwanted effects of acidosis, fatigue, and monotony. Furthermore, you will have neglected the power of your "electric" motor, and your metabolism will be like a diesel, but without the turbo. Another key to increasing your speed reserve is proper nutrition and metabolic flexibility. However, human metabolism is an ultra-precise machine, and the physiological responses within a given effort can have exponential effects beyond the linear tendencies of drift (for example, temperature). These effects may lead to sudden and dramatic changes, such as when your hybrid battery empties, and you can no longer maintain the pace. This phenomenon is simply the result of a catastrophe based on the theories founded by the French mathematician René Thom in the 1960s. The term "catastrophe" refers to the place where a function suddenly changes shape and has sudden variations (the famous butterfly effect).

POWER AND RUNNING

Increasing your speed reserve is about power, whereas force is related to the change of speed. To avoid the "catastrophe" in experiencing a decrease in speed or even abandoning the race, you must increase your safety margin in terms of power reserve. To better explain why power is crucial to running performance, we need to go into some complicated concepts. Remember, there will be a summary at the end of the chapter.

Remember that force is a product of power, and that power is the product of mass and acceleration. But it is unnecessary to become a weightlifter to increase your power reserve, instead start training using accelerations and decelerations.

It is sufficient to understand that:

- Power = Force × speed
- Force = mass × acceleration
- Acceleration = $\Delta V/\Delta t$ that is the speed variation over time

Δ is the symbol for a «change» in something.

Power is proportional to the third power (x^3) of the running speed and inversely proportional to the stride (stride length). This means that an increase in force has three times the effect on speed. Think of increasing your speed reserve as gaining a marathon safety margin and therefore, an increased power reserve. The goal is to get your muscles working at a lower percentage of their maximum power (force-speed of contraction). To achieve this, you must practice accelerations to increase power. Yes, this is exactly the opposite of many traditional marathon training books. In traditional interval training, the goal is to run at constant speeds. Old training programs are based on LSD running. We recommend against LSD running. If you do run at a constant pace, at least do it by varying stride lengths and be careful not to over-stride. One of the keys to setting your PRs is first to increase your power (speed and maximum acceleration). Once you increase your power, you will run more comfortably, have more control of your marathon speed, and better recognize and apply your optimal speed variation. You will no longer run to maintain speed but instead run to maintain a feeling of racing intensity consistent with an average effort on the marathon. The sensation of a sustained average effort is rather that of the half-marathon, on which one can apply the same race strategy. In lower distance races (10-km), we must accept to suffer as this race is both long and intense.

INCREASING SPEED RESERVE AND POWER

Sprints of 10 and 30 seconds are necessary to increase your speed reserve and marathon safety margin. It is better to have a large reserve of power than trying to maintain a high percentage of your MAS by being "enduring." To progress quickly and sustainably, rely on a training strategy that consists of increasing the limits of your power reserve. Think of your power reserve as the ability to increase your running speed at any given moment. Oxygen consumption (VO2 max) in our cells is the main reason limiting our running speed. Said another way, our reserve speed is the main reason limiting our maximum oxygen utilization. We all have a limited VO2 max for many reasons; power or muscle strength is a major limiting factor in running faster. Weak musculature limits your speed and ultimately leads to an early withdrawal from the marathon without reaching your true maximum heart rate, maximum intramuscular oxidation, and optimal lactate turnover in your muscles. Improving your metabolism is done by developing optimal power in both 10 and 30-second intervals.

Currently, most coaches prescribe training for marathons to be done "at the anaerobic threshold." We will clarify the true meaning of the anaerobic threshold and the use of MAS in your training programs. We will also reveal the meaning of these values and especially their limitations. It is preferable to have a large reserve of power rather than trying to maintain a high percentage of your MAS by running countless miles. This will save you unnecessary miles, time, and consequences in terms of chronic fatigue and injuries.

DETERMINING YOUR SPEED RESERVE

Calculating your speed reserve is something not often done by runners and coaches. Your speed reserve is simply the difference in your average marathon speed and your maximum sprint speed. If you are unable to run a top speed that is about twice that of your average marathon speed, you will start a marathon, only hoping that you can maintain the same monotonous constant speed. For example, if your average marathon speed is 15 km/hr (2 hours and

48 minutes pace) and your maximum sprint speed is 30km/hr, your speed reserve would be equal to 15 km/hr, which is 50 percent of your maximum sprint speed. We find that most runners have a speed reserve of 60 percent or greater of their maximum sprint speed.

Moreover, by increasing the speed reserve between your marathon speed (15 km/hr) and your maximum sprint speed (30 km/hr), you will be at an absolute speed equal to 15/30 = 50 percent of your maximum sprint speed rather than 15/25 = 60 percent. This will result in less neuromuscular fatigue and improve the utilization of PCr. This intramuscular super fuel allows you to have short spurts of energy and strong support for a better recoil of your elastic energy during each stride. At a 6:26 minute per mile pace (4 minutes per km), a runner takes 27,178 steps during a marathon! We understand that the average runner will struggle to reach a sprint speed double that of their average marathon pace. Still, through acceleration training, most runners can improve and increase their speed reserve.

RUNNING BIOMECHANICS

Many sports measure stride rate (cadence) to improve their efficiency. The idea of paying attention to your running cadence has only gained attention in recent years. Optimizing your cadence will give you enough power to withstand the muscular fatigue of a marathon and avoid the deterioration of your foot strike quality. An optimal foot strike is one with a short pulse time preserved beyond the 30th km. The Kenyans are well known for this. Jack Daniels famously wrote that many elites run at a cadence of 180 steps or **more** per minute. There is a lot of individual variation in strides between runners. Higher running cadences are naturally part of a minimalistic running program. While there is no magic cadence number, increasing cadence will help you finish races, avoid injury, and become more efficient.

Proper stride mechanics will increase your power reserve, which will allow you to endure a fast start and then decelerate, making small variations of speeds below the average speed and, finally, accelerating in the last 10 minutes of your marathon. Practicing accelerations and focusing on your gluteal and hamstring muscles help develop proper stride mechanics. Imagine that you are teaching your nervous system to fire and apply force in a quicker amount of time. When runners increase their cadence near the end of a marathon, this is exactly what is happening. By doing this, you can finish with a higher average speed, and better than running at a constant unbearable speed. You need a speed reserve between your marathon speed (speed zone inducing a feeling of "average" pace) and the maximum sprint speed.

This simple equation, Speed = Stride length x Stride frequency, is essential in understanding running biomechanics. In academics, we use frequency in place of rate or cadence. The cadence or frequency of our strides is nothing more than the rate at which we change foot support from one side to another. The frequency is simply the time it takes for the right foot contact to the time of the left foot contact. It merely says that to change running speed, one must either increase the distance covered (stride length) or increase your turnover (stride frequency) or some combination of the two. So, what is it when we want to run faster? It's all about power and energy. To better understand the energetics of stride and frequency, think about power as the flow of energy related to the runner's kinetic energy. Remember that we said that power is proportional to the third power (x^3) of the running speed and inversely proportional to the amplitude of the stride length. So, when we change our running speeds, it is essential to think about how it affects power. And as we shall see, it is your strength and power that determines how fast and long you can run.

ENERGY AND VO2 MAX

To determine the maximum energy at VO2 max and its associated velocity, we found that the energy at VO2 max provided more than 30 percent of the energy during a 100-m race for elite sprinters; and VO2 max provided 50 percent of the energy over a 3000-m race and only 10 percent for the marathon. However, our data only applied to mid-level marathoners (3.5 hours). Looking at Figure 19, the y-axis (vertical bar on the left) represents the contribution of energy at VO2 max in different races (x-axis) ranging from 100 meters to the marathon. It is amazing to think that the energy spent at VO2 max for a marathon represents only 10 percent of the total energy expended during a marathon. This may seem surprising, knowing that we run at 65 – 80 percent of our VO2 max in terms of power demand.

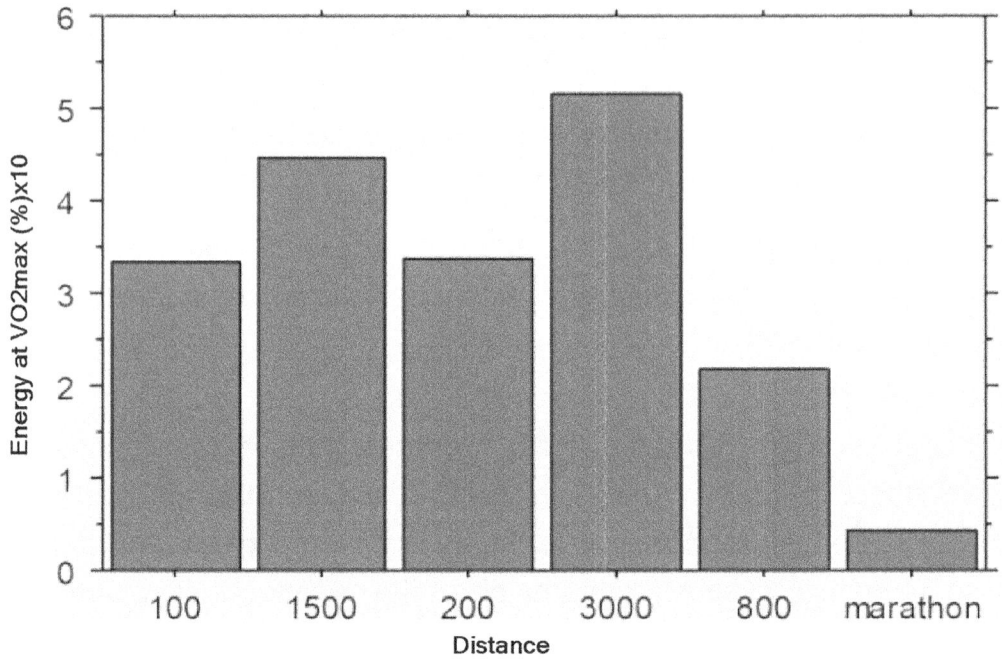

Figure 19. Contribution of energy to VO2 max as a function of the total energy required (in %) in different track and field events (Molinari 2018).

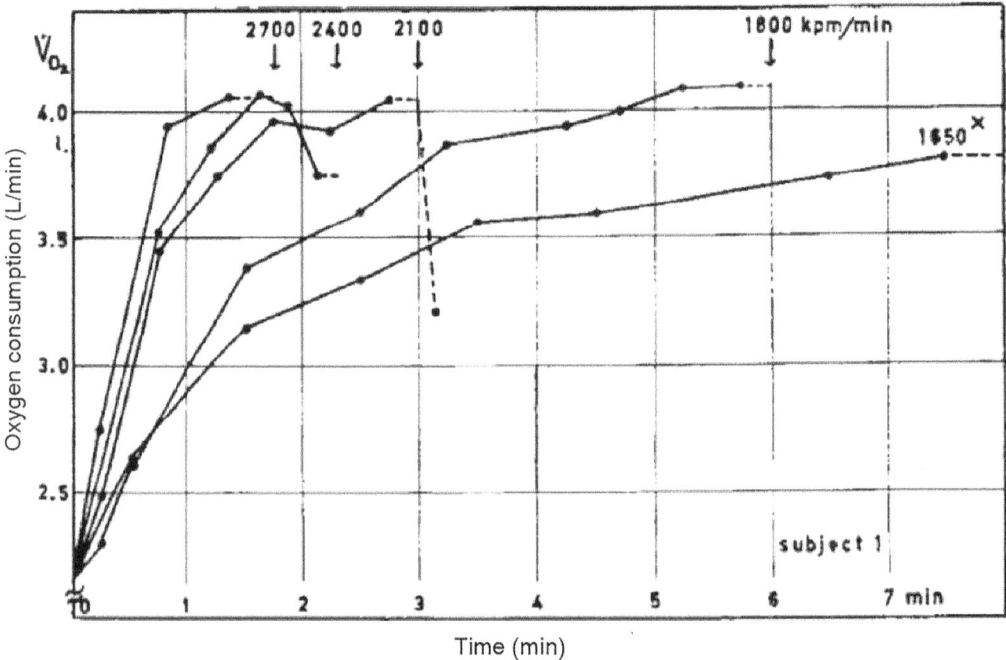

Figure 20. In 1961, Astrand and Saltin, the masters of the magnificent Swedish school of physiology, had already demonstrated in 1961 that VO2 max could be reached in less than 3 minutes starting from rest (Astrand and Saltin 1961).

Since we can reach VO2 max seconds after a strong acceleration, our bodies automatically stop exercise at VO2 max; this is caused by:

- The perception of pain resulting from a significant shortness of breath or muscular pain.

- Due to neural fatigue or the inability to sustain power.

- Due to a decrease in cadence or muscle strength even with direct neuromuscular stimulation.

Cardiac function is not the limiting factor. We can reach VO2 max and maximum heart rate (HR max) by varying the power output. In this configuration, it is possible to maintain VO2 max for more than 25 minutes. We can assume that it is possible to maintain VO2 max even longer if we know the variation of power (velocity). The advantage of providing (long) energy for VO2 max is to create the possibility of producing adenosine-tri-phosphate (ATP) without accumulating intracellular acid beyond the possibilities of its elimination, but also, to recycle lactate and to reconstitute mitochondrial PCr (our two electric batteries).

When a top sprinter runs 100-m at his absolute maximum, he will be at VO2 max. Similarly, research has shown that an elite sprinter must have a minimum VO2 max of 55 ml/min/kg. In marathons, we have seen previously that the elite races are won with U-shaped patterns (convex), with a fast start, a tendency to run more distance at speeds below the average speed, and finishing with a strong acceleration for about 2 km.

PERFORMANCE ARISES FROM COOPERATION IN DIVERSITY

Nature always reminds us when we try to manipulate and control a single piece of our metabolism. Varying the speed during training and competition stimulates the development of PCr/Cr shuttles in the slow-twitch muscles and an increase in the synthesis of mitochondria, optimizing the ability to regenerate PCr. Therefore, it is necessary to integrate acceleration phases in training (more critical than speedwork alone) to partially deplete PCr, which is a signal of increased oxygen consumption. This same oxygen consumption allows the PCr shuttle to function at high rates. But this only happens when the PCr shuttle stabilizes after a few sets of speed variations. You will also be able to recruit more muscle fibers, including the intermediate muscle fibers (slow/fast), which will be activated at lower relative tensions levels than slow fibers. **It is important to consider this system as the cooperation between all our muscular fibers and all our metabolisms without compartmentalizing metabolic systems and single types of muscle fibers.** Thus, during the acceleration phases, the fast fibers can develop this shuttle system while retaining their specificity.

In sprinters, we saw that the energy at VO2 max represented more than 30 percent of the energy supply over 100-m. In a way, we can say that Usain Bolt was more robust thanks to his estimated VO2 max of 66 ml/min/kg according to his 400-m performances as a junior (47.12 seconds). Practicing several sports and disciplines from a young age and throughout life stimulates this muscle fiber diversity. It is also important to reference the forty-year-old who can run 400-m in 45.28 seconds and the fifty-nine-year-old who can run a 2:31 marathon. They both have a VO2 max of 68 ml/min/kg and can finish a marathon in less than 3 hours. These runners exemplify the importance of building a strong power/speed reserve. With such a power reserve, they can use it to vary the speed, resulting in less fatigue and recovery time, and a higher average speed than they would have achieved otherwise running at a constant speed or pace. Aerobics and sprints are not incompatible; it is quite the opposite. Developing your aerobic engine is necessary to optimize your ability to perform longer and faster sprint repetitions. In the sport of soccer (football in Europe), this is what allows team sports specialists to develop more impactful accelerations in the second half of the game.

Finally, rather than considering the "three energy metabolisms" separately, we should rather speak of an energetic continuum since the utilization of our glucose and fat reserves change according to the intensity of the race. Mitochondrial respiration stimulates PCr/Cr shuttles to resynthesize PCr stores at the cellular level of muscle contractile proteins (Figure 21). The different types of training in terms of intensity and duration, activate the reaction rates of these different stages, and never specifically a single metabolic pathway. Incorporating sprints (accelerations) with short recovery times makes it possible to develop the aerobic system. Thus, the regeneration of PCr via the shuttle system between the mitochondrial production of ATP and the contractile muscle proteins.

Acceleration is, therefore, key to effective training to increase your power reserve for the marathon.

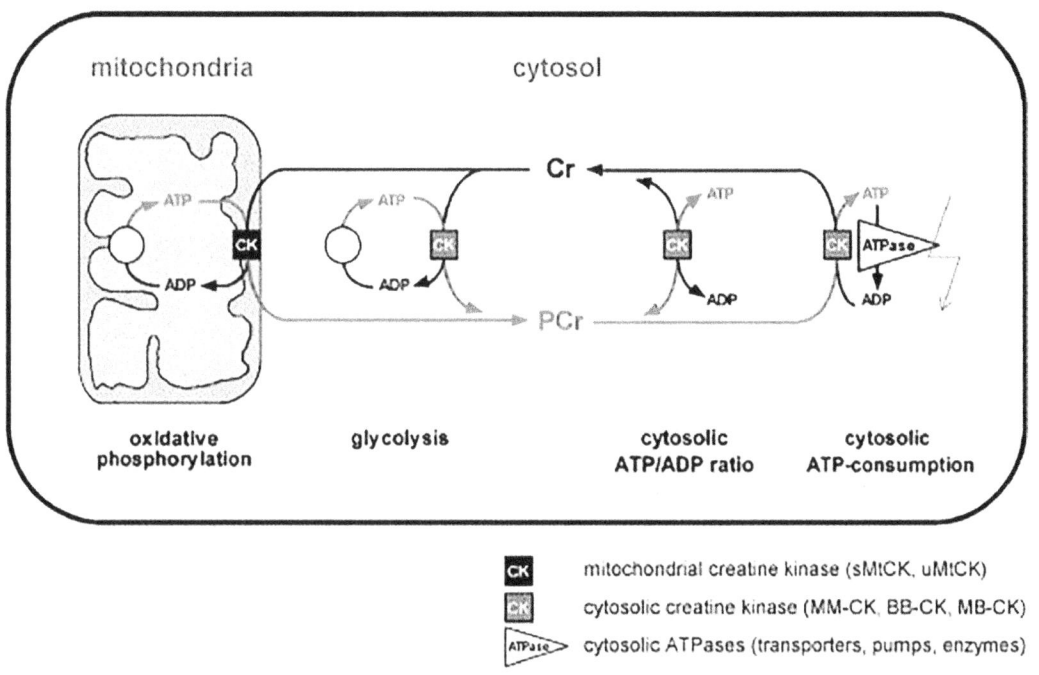

Figure 21. The action of Creatine Kinase/Phosphocreatine (CK/PCr) shuttles by cascade. Oxidative phosphorylation is the process of phosphorylation of adenosine-di-phosphate (ADP) into ATP through the energy released by the oxidation of electron donors in the respiratory chain (Schlattner 2006).

THE ESSENTIAL ROLE OF LACTATE

Lactate is another type of sugar and is essential in allowing us to accelerate. The reason is that lactate combines with hydrogen ions via aerobic metabolism during an effort. In this example, lactate is a capacitor (the ability of a system to store an electric charge) as we previously explained, a kind of recyclable sugar energy stock at any point of the race when you slow down slightly below the average speed. Recall that it is possible to quickly reach VO2 max, (in a few seconds) when we produce strong accelerations. By accelerating, we unload our electric battery, the PCr shuttle, activating a rise in oxygen consumption, which increases the oxidation of carbohydrates (Francescato 2008). A fast race start is important because it uses our PCr reserves to quickly reach a high level of VO2, increasing the concentration of blood lactate. Then as we slow down, the PCr stores are replenished, and the lactate concentration stabilizes. Lactate is beneficial because it supports further accelerations by trapping hydrogen (H +) ions. Without lactate, the hydrogen ions would increase too much and result in a decrease in blood pH and increase muscle acidosis.

Redox reactions and the role of nicotinamide-adenine-dinucleotide (NADH)

When a molecule accepts electrons from an electron donor, it is said to be "reduced," when a molecule gives its electrons to another molecule, it is an "oxidation" reaction. A useful way to remember this is OIL RIG: oxidation loses electrons, reduction gains electrons. Redox reactions are always coupled. In other words, one molecule cannot be reduced without another first being oxidized. The molecule that gives its electrons is called an oxidizing agent, while a molecule that accepts electrons is a reducing agent. The oxidation phenomenon does not necessarily imply oxygen. However, the term oxidation comes from the fact that oxygen is the quintessential reducer and tends to accept electrons. Thus, oxygen is an extraordinarily strong oxidizing agent. During aerobic metabolism, cells use this property of oxygen as the final acceptor of electrons at the end of the respiratory chain. Two molecules also play an important role in these oxidation-reduction reactions, namely Nicotinamide Adenine Dinucleotide (NAD) and Flavin Adenine Dinucleotide (FAD). Each molecule of NAD and FAD can accept two electrons according to the reversible reactions: $FAD + 2 H^+ \leftrightarrow FADH + H^+$ and $NAD + 2 H^+ \leftrightarrow NADH + H^+$. It is important to realize that all of this happens in the mitochondria. About the NADH shuttle in mitochondria: The NADH generated during glycolysis must be converted back into NAD so that glycolysis continues (this happens in the second part of glycolysis). The conversion of NADH into NAD can be done when the pyruvic acid accepts the hydrogen protons (H+) to form lactate. However, during aerobic metabolism and when glycolysis is not so fast that it overwhelms mitochondrial

> respiratory chain, the conversion of NADH into NAD can be carried out by the NADH shuttle through the mitochondrial membrane. The NADH then places its hydrogens into the mitochondria where the electron transport chain is taking place, and the H+ combines with oxygen to form water and carbon dioxide.

Raising the lactate concentration serves a second purpose by signaling to the muscle cell that it needs to increase its oxygen uptake. Training improves this sensitivity of oxidative phosphorylation to lactate (more precisely, the increase of protons and the NADH/NAD ratio). This is why training lowers the lactate concentration at a given speed, signifying higher sensitivity of the respiratory chain to the lactate concentration. Training improves the transmission of information in the cell, and we are far from having approached the subtleties of the activation and signaling pathways that are discovered each year (Gibala 2012).

High-Intensity Interval Training (HIIT) training is fashionable and has recently appeared in many research articles. However, it still needs to be revolutionized, especially when it comes to marathon training. Indeed, HIIT training's effectiveness is proven, but it is difficult to highlight in a customized protocol. This is partly because scientific publications have difficulty thinking of training as being related to the person's physiological profile. Before giving you the keys to this interval/acceleration training protocol (the productive part of the HIIT is the deceleration), we will clarify the concept of acceleration. Thus, it is necessary to increase its maximum power and its force and frequency (velocity) at high speeds (acceleration). Remember that force is defined as the product of mass by acceleration according to Newton's second law:

$$F = m \times a$$

where F is the force in Newtons, m is the mass in kg, and a is the acceleration in m/s^2. One Newton is the force needed to accelerate a mass of 1 kg of 1 m/s^2.

Muscular strength is an underemphasized area of marathon training. Muscular strength is an essential component of energy efficiency that works by establishing elastic energy to the foot on the ground. This is the energy keeping you from "dropping to the ground" at mile twenty of a marathon and forcing you to double your efforts to maintain speed. In terms of work capacity, marathon runners have a very narrow focus. If we think of muscular strength or work as the amount of energy expended over time, a runner has a meager output compared to that of a sprinter or CrossFit athlete. Endurance runners do not put in a lot of effort into building their upper body strength or gluteal muscles. If we want to maintain our efficiency while running, we should consider investing in strengthening our other muscle groups. Practicing things like squats, deadlifts, and upper body exercises will increase our overall strength and increase the area under the curve of our work capacity.

An excellent example is those runners who cannot continue a marathon due to back pain. Developing good gluteal and spinal muscle strength ensures that back pain will be less of a factor during a long marathon. These muscle groups will not develop only through running; some cross-training is necessary. Every runner must find their balance as to how much they want to develop other areas, but the critical thing to realize is that strength is a key element of energy efficiency.

The famous "anaerobic threshold velocity" is only a short, stepwise increasing rate protocol (1–3 minutes). MAS fits in the same category. It must be kept in mind that time is the "second guest" of the race and cannot be dissociated from speed. Ann Snyder (1993) researched overtraining, and she observed that the best way to avoid overtraining was to vary the speed and intensity in training. The most efficient way to increase power reserve is to increase the force by accelerating on a flat surface and then a slope of less than 8 percent or a very slight slope with a load of 5 percent of the body weight. Since Force = mass × acceleration, according to Newton's second law of mechanics, we must plan our accelerations with respect to the mass components of force. Classical 30-30s training or longer intervals (3-minutes) are traumatic as runners increase their speeds abruptly (about ten times faster than on a "strong" acceleration) and then try to maintain these high speeds at all costs. Although these interval/intermittent workouts affect all metabolisms, a deductive reasoning (a priori) approach to increasing intensity and duration is risky. Through experience and observation, we created a new training protocol in our outside laboratory using acceleration training. We first verified this notion of acceleration training in animal models and then finally with numerous runners providing us possible answers to the limits of the protocols described earlier.

THREE DIFFERENT TYPES OF ACCELERATIONS

Acceleration training is based on a sequence of three different types of accelerations (Figure 22). Sometimes, these are called progression runs. Each acceleration is performed to exhaustion and interspersed with a rest of 30 minutes. The first acceleration starts gently (interpreted arbitrarily by the individual). The second acceleration increases more abruptly, and the third is short and intense. It is difficult for a human to feel/control his speed without an indicator (just as it is difficult to say how fast we run or how fast a car rolls). However, a human can perfectly feel and control accelerations or decelerations. Thus, it is possible to ask a person to increase (slightly/moderately/intensively) his/her running speed until exhaustion. The significant advantage of this type of training is the possibility of performing this type of training without equipment. Individualization is self-realized, and we can regulate our acceleration to sensations on simple "soft, medium, or strong" acceleration instructions.

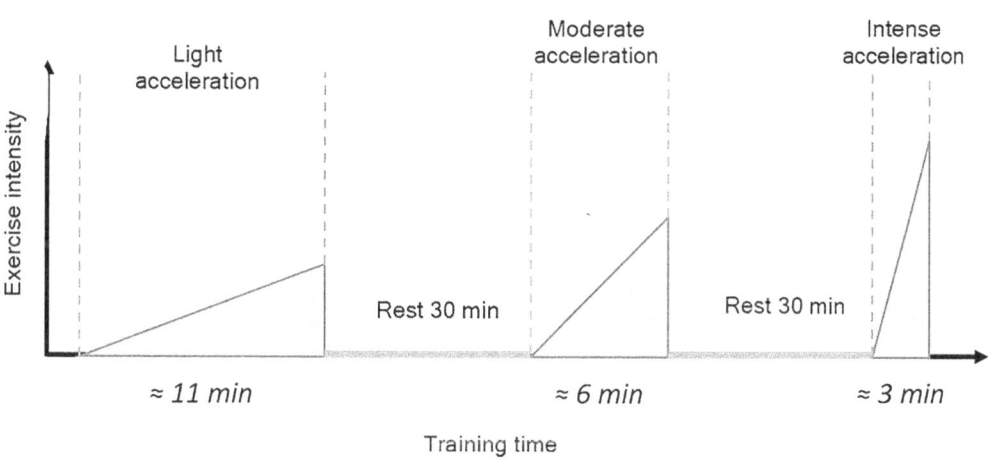

Figure 22. These tests were performed in humans and found that each subject took the same amount of time to reach exhaustion in each acceleration. Approximately 11 minutes for a light acceleration; 6 minutes for a moderate acceleration; and 3 minutes for a strong acceleration (Billat 2018).

In our studies, we found that constant accelerations produced the best results. Because of the similarities with intermittent training (reaching maximum exercise intensities, speed variations), this training stimulates all metabolisms in various ways, keeping exercise fun and self-directed. On the other hand, unlike intermittent workouts, this new workout protocol does not abruptly reach the maximum exercise intensities, but gradually and without muscle or joint trauma. This is important, especially for inexperienced and older runners. Finally, the goal is to produce an improvement in the quality of the muscular force, which is defined as the acceleration of a mass. By working accelerations, this allows a natural improvement of the quality of the muscular force. Acceleration training, therefore, has many advantages while limiting the disadvantages.

Our abilities to regulate strength and acceleration are natural, whereas it is difficult for us to maintain a constant speed without a reference. This is logical since we feel the forces and the force components. Remember that force = mass × acceleration according to Newton's second law of mechanics. We can follow setpoints (external or internal) of constant accelerations at different values, which naturally points us in a stable physiological state by the variation of speed and not by its constancy. By adjusting our accelerations, we will learn to be more accurate as we will create a broad speed range (the famous power/speed reserve). We have worked with numerous athletes and provided them with simple acceleration instructions, resulting in the beneficial effects of this type of training. It is effective, fun, and self-managed without going beyond one's limits by always trying to maintain a constant speed. All this does not happen at once, as everything is a process. For example, as soon as you feel that you can no longer accelerate, you should stop it.

Interestingly, we can give simple instructions of feeling the sensation of accelerations (mild, medium, and strong) and obtain a perfect constant acceleration until exhaustion. Small catch-up effects are visible on the graphs, but the goal is to obtain a linear increase of speed as a function of time and this, at three distinct levels of acceleration. In a group of ten runners (with small individual differences), the average value of perceived accelerations ranged from mild to strong, in a group of marathon runners at three-hours and forty-minutes.

For those academically inclined, we can use an equation describing constant acceleration to examine the relationship between the distance traveled as a function of time assuming we are constantly accelerating:

$$d = \tfrac{1}{2} at^2$$

where d is the running distance in meters, a is the acceleration in m/s², and t is the running time in seconds. This just shows that average acceleration is about twice that of the mild, and the strong acceleration was double the average. These types of equations are used to calculate the maximum distances possible to run with a given acceleration.

ACCELERATING IS NATURAL – NEURAL GRID CELLS

We have grid cells in our brain that allow us to know our position in space, which is why we can detect accelerations and decelerations without a reference. During a race, it has been shown that in the absence of external dynamic signals, the grid cells in the brain incorporate self-generated distance and time information to encode a representation of the experiment (Krause 2015). This agrees with our discovery that a runner (even inexperienced) can control their accelerations without external cues by the relation between distance and time elapsed.

A grid cell is a type of neuron present in the brain that allows one to know their position in space. The grid cells get their name from the fact that by connecting the centers of their activation fields, we get a triangular grid. The grid cells were discovered in 2005 by Edvard Moser. He won the Nobel Prize in Physiology/Medicine for the discovery of grid cells constituting a positioning system in the brain. The arrangement of the spatial activation fields of the grid cells shows an equal distance between each neighboring cell. This observation led to the hypothesis that these cells encode a cognitive representation of Euclidean-type space. The discovery also suggests a dynamic position computation mechanism based on continuously updated information about position and direction.

The question is to correctly describe the speed curve as a function of the runner's time, which accelerates without any external clues. We showed that a runner controls his speed every four seconds with a recall capacity to keep the acceleration constant. Indeed, what controls this mechanism has yet to be identified. Nevertheless, we have shown that it could be related to the race distance. The acceleration corrections are such that the race distance is almost deterministic if the acceleration were constant. While it is well known that runners can adapt their speed to achieve specific goals and performance, this is the first time that the control of self-paced accelerations during running tests has been demonstrated. This work suggests that we may be programming our accelerations more than our speeds as it is difficult for humans to maintain a constant speed, as we are not robots. Since we proceed by pulse which is defined as the application of a propulsive force to the ground for a certain period. We feel the muscular forces at play and recall again that the force is defined as the ability to accelerate a mass (a force of 1 Newton is the force needed to accelerate a mass of 1 kg of 1 m/s^2). This discovery can be a significant element in the search for the optimal variation of the race speed to stimulate the body and adapt it to new forces and impulses (training objective) in competition. However, we still do not know which control variables determine these optimal variations for the time being.

CHAPTER 6 SUMMARY

CONCEPT: Human metabolism is an ultra-precise machine, and the physiological responses within a given effort can have exponential effects beyond the linear tendencies of drift (for example, temperature). These effects may lead to sudden and dramatic changes, such as when your hybrid battery empties, and you can no longer maintain the pace. This phenomenon is simply the result of a "catastrophe." Increasing your speed reserve is all about power and force is related to the change of speed. To avoid the "catastrophe" in the sense of experiencing a decrease in speed or even abandoning the race, you must increase your safety margin in terms of power reserve.

APPLICATION: You must increase your speed reserve to run your marathon without cracking and with all the pleasure of running it below your average speed for over half of the race. Running a marathon using speed variations is the key to finishing the event and enjoying the experience. If you train using traditional lactate thresholds, you will never succeed in being able to vary your speed in a marathon. Running at the same speeds will induce the harmful effects of acidosis, fatigue, and monotony. Indeed, you will have neglected the power of your "electric" motor, and your metabolism will be like a diesel, but without the turbo. Another key to increasing your speed reserve is proper nutrition and metabolic flexibility. If you are unable to achieve a top speed that is about twice that of your average marathon speed, you will take the start every time, hoping that you can maintain the same monotonous constant speed.

CHAPTER 7

VARIABLE SPEED ACCELERATION TRAINING

Variable speed acceleration training improves VO2 max and efficiency. It is natural to perform and beneficial in elite runners, animal models, and even our elderly population. The book, *Running with the Kenyans*, describes how some of the world's best runners don't use sophisticated training watches; instead, they practice accelerations. Haile Gebrselassie is known for not using multiphase periodization training schedules. Rather, he performs long runs using his sensations and chooses the distances that give him the most confidence going into a marathon. He does not perform 200 or 400-m intervals as he knows that type of training will lead to injury. Many successful training programs employ acceleration training. In marathon running, switching gears to take the lead, or put in a final kick demands an increase in pace, can be the difference between winning and losing. Accelerating up a hill is often the difference between efficiently going up a hill versus struggling to maintain pace and form.

REAL-LIFE EXAMPLES OF ACCELERATION-BASED TRAINING

Brenda Martinez is a well-known American Track & Field runner and represented team USA in the 2016 Olympic games. She earned a silver medal at the 2013 IAAF World Championships in the 800-m race and set a world record in the Distance Medley Relay in 2015. Brenda's coach and husband, Carlos Handler, had her run Billat 30-30s twice a week and said, "they certainly work!" He felt that the 30-30s benefited Brenda by helping her increase fitness quickly without the stress of focusing on hitting specific times during in an interval or on the track. She also performed the Rabit test and likes the idea of practicing running to her sensations. Brenda had to sit out the 2019 season due to injury, so she and her coach were motivated to try acceleration-based workouts that could limit her risk of injuries. Currently, Brenda is working to qualify for the 2021 Olympic Games in Tokyo.

Theresa Hailey, recently qualified for the 2020 USA Olympic Marathon trials and was the winner of the 2013 Vancouver USA Half Marathon and loves the Billat intervals. She ran a PB of 2:44:19 at the CIM marathon in 2017. Focusing on shorter events, she performed four weeks of Billat 30-30s (version 2), shortly after she ran a 10-km PB of 34:52. Two months later, still utilizing the acceleration-based workouts, she posted a 3-km PB of 9:42:27, 5-km PB of 16:46, and 1600-m PB of 4:50:61 all within a twenty-one-day window. Theresa was quoted saying that performing the Billat workouts "pushed me to run in an uncomfortable zone but without the pressure. I loved that it was up to me to choose when to stop, but at the same time, it tested me both mentally and physically." Each time she performed the workouts, her splits began to decrease, which boosted her confidence. She looked forward to each workout. Once she found the Billat workouts' rhythm, she had complete control over each speed zone, and how hard she pushed was entirely up to her. She gained confidence and became more competitive after going through a Billat cycle of training.

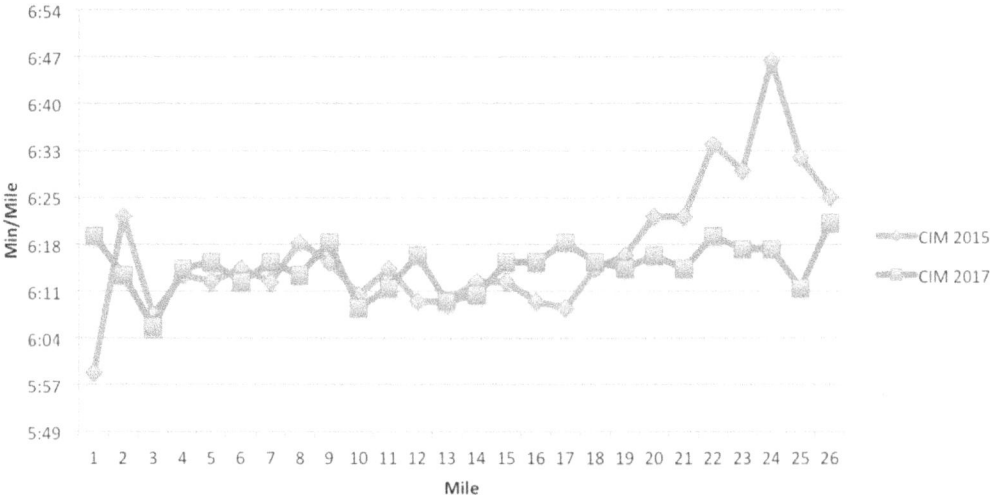

Figure 23. Theresa Hailey's CIM USA Olympic qualifying marathon races. Comparing the 2015 race to the 2017 race, one can see that she had a fast start in 2017, ran with variable speed oscillations, and finished fast in the final kilometers. In 2015, she cracked by mile 17, and her pace dropped considerably.

ACCELERATION BASED VERSUS CONSTANT PACED TRAINING

An interesting experiment is to go out and free-run a 10-km, and then measure your average pace using your GPS-watch. Then run that same distance, but at a constant pace, with the same average speed, and you will find that in most cases, you will only be able to hold that pace for about 7000-m. Dr. Billat showed this in a 2006 research paper; the free-running group ran at about a 5 percent lower VO2 than the constant pace group, speed variations were higher in the free-running group, and the free-running group spent 10 percent less time at VO2 max. Lactate measurements at the threshold and the end of 10,000 meters were both lower in the free-running group versus the constant pace running group. This research highlights the advantages of variable pace running, allowing the runner's metabolism to work between anaerobic and aerobic glycolysis efficiently and allowing the recycling of lactate and creatine phosphate synthesis. Many runners choose a cadence that gives comfort, but not necessarily the best race economy. Most race strategies are not going to help us in a real race situation since we are trying to get from point A to point B in as little time as possible. We are not machines with control loops in anticipatory action (predictive control or feed-forward). Hopefully, you can see that there are other ways to train for the marathon.

In another research paper, our laboratory wanted to answer whether acceleration-based training was better than constant paced training (Launay 2017). We had senescent mice (equivalent to eighty human years) perform endurance training based on variable accelerations or constant pace at eighty percent of their MAS. We found that varied acceleration training leads to better adaptations of both anaerobic and aerobic metabolisms, mainly because of the higher intensity of exercise. Varied accelerating training is an integral part of the BillaTraining.com program, and we have shown that it has positive impacts on antioxidant defense systems, insulin sensitivity, and protein turnover. We have helped improve the lives of many older runners using these techniques. An excellent real-life example of using varied acceleration training to improve VO2 max is our centenarian athlete Robert Marchand. We were able to improve Robert's VO2 max even beyond his hundredth birthday. Since longevity is tightly connected to VO2 max, so in this sense, we have improved his performance and longevity.

IMPROVING VO2 MAX AT ANY AGE

We have demonstrated that humans can improve VO2 max and peak power at any age (Billat 2017). In contrast, low-intensity endurance training develops anaerobic metabolism poorly. Having a good anaerobic metabolism is essential in marathon running and quality of life since it is essential to vary the race's speed. Interval-based training does not allow for the optimal development of physiological adaptations as compared to varied acceleration training. The goal of classic intervals is to maintain a high-intensity speed resulting in exhaustion; in contrast, acceleration-based training is not. Acceleration-based training has the dual benefit of continuous training and interval training. It stimulates the body without exhaustion, saving time, and preventing injuries. Besides, given the need to promote exercise among seniors, a short-term acceleration training programs increase their motivation. Varied acceleration training is what our human bodies are ultimately designed to perform.

Research suggests that in just two weeks of training (two 20-minute sessions per week), varied acceleration training allows one to increase power superior to endurance training (five 60-minute sessions per week) (Niel 2017). This study's results are impressive if we judge the gain in performance and VO2 max, especially considering the training duration of only two weeks. Studies in mice have shown some interesting results highlighting the differences between varied acceleration training to endurance training. Indeed, humans are more complex than mice, but we can learn from the results. Over two weeks, one group of mice performed constant endurance training, the other group of mice acceleration training. Many important differences exist when comparing the mice who completed 20 endurance training sessions to mice who completed just 5 sessions of acceleration training.

If we look at the differences between one session of acceleration training:

- 3.3 times less running time
- 2.8 times less distance
- 1.28 higher average speed
- 2.8 times higher maximum exercise intensity

Now if we compare the differences in the total sessions:

- 12.7 times less running time for the acceleration training group
- 7.6 times less distance to travel for the accelerating training group
- A 1.25-fold average session speed for acceleration training group
- A maximum exercise intensity 2.9 times higher for acceleration training group

In summary, you can spend a lot less time training, decrease the risk of injury, decrease the risk of overtraining, and receive the same benefits. In other studies of acceleration training in an aged mouse model, we showed large differences in performance improvements in peak speeds. This is exciting because it shows that with even a small amount of acceleration training, we can improve our VO2 max. With the training, every mouse was able to improve their accelerations as well as their peak speeds. It is important to remember that these aged mice are the equivalent of eighty-years in humans. The mice in the endurance group showed a decrease in their performance between the pre and post-test at 4 weeks. No changes were detected for the control group. In all tests, VO2 max was measured, but no significant changes were observed in any of the groups. This shows that VO2 max is not immediately sensitive to training and is not necessary to the increase in exercise performance (Vpeak and support time limit). In other words, it is not necessary to change VO2 max to see an increase in performance.

Increasing VO2 max at Any Age – Robert Marchand

Robert Marchand – One-hundred-and-six-year old cyclist and world record holder

Regular exercise positively enhances the health and independence in people who live past one hundred years of age (centenarians). But only recently, have direct assessments of centenarians been performed in laboratories. Enter one-hundred-and-six-year-old French cyclist, Robert Marchand. He has been cycling for an exceptionally long time. Racing semi-professionally in his twenties, and only returning to cycling in his sixties, he participated in several major races, including Bordeaux to Paris and Paris to Roubaix. In 1992, he cycled from Paris to Moscow. Since his one-hundredth birthday, he has been followed closely in Dr. Billat's research lab. At one-hundred-and-one years old, he held the one-hour cycling record for the hundred-plus category. In 2017, he set the one-hour cycling record in the one-hundred-and-five-year old plus age group, covering 22.5 km (14 miles) in one hour. At the age of one-hundred-and-five-years old, he was recognized as the world's oldest competitive cyclist by the Guinness World Records. His performance and metrics were studied for the next several years. He performed tests on the cycling ergometer to determine heart rate, VO2 max, and power. He trains using the 80/20 rule, 80 percent low intensity, 20 percent higher intensity. He cycles about 5000-km (3000 miles) per year. Very importantly, he has been able to keep his muscle mass and weight about the same. Ultimately, he was able to increase his VO2 max to 40 ml/kg/min, his max heart rate in the 130s, and his power increased from 90 to 125 watts.

Not There to Win, But to Increase Vitality

Robert Marchand wanted to increase his VO2 to add quality and vitality to his current life, rather than avoid death. Robert Marchand's experience is vital for many reasons. Participation and performance in the masters' groups are increasing. Many people are self-engineering bio-optimization regimens to increase longevity. We don't have a lot of experience with so-called "very old masters athletes." For example, among octogenarian athletes, new VO2 max records are set and comparable to the average human in their forties. Marchand's VO2 max is the same as a man half his age who has a sedentary lifestyle. Marchand's essential qualities are that he has a large oxygen consumption thanks to an exceptional heart, the ability to reach a high heart rate, and an exceptional VO2 max for his age.

Marchand's Workout Routine

He varies his accelerations on the bicycle between 60 and 85 RPM and reaches a max heart rate in the 130s. He uses resistance bands and performs pushups. Moreover, as he ages, Marchand's philosophy is never to lose sight of an essential goal: to keep his muscles working. He rides every day on his home trainer and outside with his Paris cycling club L'Ardechois when the weather permits.

Muscle Loss - Accelerated Sarcopenia

We cannot ignore the part of Robert Marchand's story, where he needed to be persuaded by his doctors to take up eating protein again. For personal reasons, Marchand veered away from his dietary recommendations and gave up eating meat one month before his world record attempt. He was protesting about how animals are mistreated in the factory production process. Certainly justified, but unfortunately, as Marchand's protein intake decreased, he quickly lost muscle mass, and his performance suffered. For the hour record challenge, he measured 1.50 meters tall (4 feet 11 inches) and weighing just 50 kg (110 pounds). He also blamed missing his 10-minute warning at the end of the event to not eating correctly. Three years earlier, during his hour record challenge, he rode an additional 4.3 km (or about 2.6 miles).

His rapid decline in muscle mass suggests that he experienced "accelerated sarcopenia." Protein intake and muscle mass contribute significantly to VO2 max and power output and, ultimately, vitality, especially in a one-hundred-and-five-year-old human. There is no easy answer to this question, but Robert Marchand's physiology suffered from not eating a rich protein source for just thirty days. Dr. Billat probably knows more about how Marchand's body works than anyone. She also noted that his lack of protein affected his muscle mass. It is worth noting that it is possible to eat enough protein on a vegetarian diet (especially with eggs), but it is difficult without adequate knowledge and resources. Marchand's diet is limited due to budget, and consuming quality meats could be difficult on such a budget. This also highlights a scenario unique to centenarians. If you live to one hundred, you are highly likely to outlive your retirement!

Robert Marchand's Secret - Home Life and Optimism

According to Dr. Veronique Billat, Robert Marchand lives alone in his Parisian studio flat, but he is sustained by optimism, laughter, and many friends. Also, his natural curiosity and astonishment keep him going, according to his friends. He eats "a la française," which means that he eats a simple French regime. Marchand does not count calories or the amount of protein he consumes each day. He just eats as he feels. Again, the French, as a culture, dislike counting anything or limiting what they

> can eat. Just like children are very in tune with their satiety centers, most French people are as well. When he is done eating, he simply stops.
>
> - Morning - He eats a typical French breakfast, some fruit, full-fat yogurt, French bread, and coffee. As is common in French culture, he walks to the boulangerie (bread shop) each day and buys a fresh baguette.
> - Afternoon - He eats a serving of chicken, sardines, mackerel in oil, or eggs and mushrooms, along with green beans and perhaps some bread.
> - Night - Most nights, he eats a bowl of soup, some cheese, and some wine. This could be typical for many older people, as most centenarians look for simple ways to prepare meals.
>
> After his one-hundred-and-sixth birthday, Marchand's doctors advised him against competing for any more world records. He "retired," but he is still racing and riding. He recently competed in a 4000-m Velodrome race in Paris. Marchand can be quoted saying, "C'est moi qui decide et je veux rouler" (I'm the one that decides, and I want to ride). According to Marchand, he intends to keep pedaling as long as he can stretch his legs. Marchand's inspirational approach to life and healthy living has already won the world over.

In conclusion, we can say that acceleration-based training is advantageous because each session is short; the gains are substantial in a short time. Five sessions over two weeks with a total exercise time of 1 hour and 36 minutes was all it took to see benefits in our animal model. We have seen the benefits of acceleration training in our athletes for years. Also, acceleration-based training does not require intricate knowledge of the lower level of VO2 max or MAS. It is enough for someone to accelerate to easy, medium, and hard sensations. In humans, this is easy to achieve, and no electronic gadgets are required. Humans are perfectly hard-wired to perceive constant accelerations at three levels of intensity. This effectiveness of accelerating training includes a whole range of exercise intensities (from low intensity to high intensity), stimulating the various pathways of energy metabolism, without however having to exercise at high intensities that completely exhaust the runner. Indeed, the advantage of the acceleration training is this smooth rise in speed as a function of time, unlike interval training, which often involves sudden accelerations. In the next chapter, we will show you how to apply these principals of acceleration-based training to your workouts and training routines.

CHAPTER 7 SUMMARY

CONCEPT: Variable speed acceleration training improves VO2 max and efficiency. It is natural to perform and can be used in all runners, animal models, and even our elderly population. In marathon running, switching gears to take the lead, or putting in a final kick demands an increase in pace, which can sometimes be the difference between winning and losing. Accelerating up a hill is often the difference between efficiently going up a hill versus struggling to maintain pace and form. Many successful training programs employ acceleration training.

APPLICATION: Theresa Hailey practices acceleration-based intervals. She performed four weeks of Billat 30-30s (version 2), shortly after she ran a 10-km PB of 34:52. Two months later, still utilizing the acceleration-based workouts, she posted a 3-km PB of 9:42:27, 5km PB of 16:46, and 1600-m PB of 4:50:61 all within a twenty-one-day window. Once she found the rhythm of the Billat workouts, she had complete control over each speed zone, and how fast she pushed was entirely up to her. She gained confidence and became more competitive. Haile Gebrselassie is known for not using multiphase periodization training schedules. Instead, he performs runs by feel and does the workouts that give him the most confidence going into a marathon. He does not perform 200 or 400-m intervals. He knows that type of training will lead to injury.

CHAPTER 8

ACCELERATION BASED TRAINING – BIOCHEMISTRY, ENZYMES, AND LACTATE

LACTATE IN ACCELERATION TRAINING VERSUS ENDURANCE TRAINING

EVERY ENDURANCE ATHLETE IS LOOKING for workouts to gain fitness quickly. If you are looking for so-called "magic bullets," lactate training is one place to start. It is crucial to think of lactate as a friend and not a foe! As discussed earlier, lactate is shuttled from active muscles to less active muscles. These less active muscle groups are are better oxygenated, and can use lactate for energy, thereby sparing glycogen. It is important to train this shuttle to be better able to use lactate as energy. The idea is to repeat certain intervals to ramp up your metabolism to something close to VO2 max and hold it long enough to improve your aerobic capacity. We have found this type of training superior to long anaerobic intervals; the benefits of these exercises are at MAS and the fluctuation of blood lactate levels. Anytime you are at MAS, this is where the magic happens, and your body adapts. When we run hard and then slow down, we continue breathing hard for some time afterward. Exercise physiologists used to call this "oxygen debt," but we now know that oxygen has nothing to do with it.

As you may recall, our muscles need ATP to break the bonds between actin and myosin in the muscle fibrils and relax the muscle. This "oxygen debt" is, in fact, a disruption of homeostasis involving ATP regeneration. Restoration of high-energy molecules like ATP and PCr takes only milliseconds in the muscle cells. During these fast-paced recoveries, the body is working to adapt to the excess lactate. This is why the brain, heart, muscles, and diaphragm adapt to using lactate for fuel rather than stealing glucose from your larger hard-working muscles like the quadriceps and gluteus muscles. Recall that lactate is an integral part of our hybrid electric motors. The acceleration group showed an increase in blood lactate during the post-test, while the endurance group showed a decrease in post-training blood lactate. Even though both results coincide with performance gains, the differences in blood lactate are important.

> ### Lactate and Lactic Acid
>
> You have undoubtedly heard your coach or trainer use the word "lactic acid" and "lactate" interchangeably. Many believe these two things are the same, but they are quite different. We understand that the term "lactic acid" has been used in practice for over one hundred years. There is no such entity as lactic acid in any human cell or physiological system. It is impossible, based on the fundamental laws of physics that underpin biochemistry, physiology, or acid-base chemistry. Cells present in living systems are regulated between a pH of 6.0 and 7.45.

Lactate is produced by your body in response to aerobic exercise and serves as a fuel to muscles and especially the heart. During exercise, you are using oxygen at higher rates. As you know, the body is always using aerobic and anaerobic metabolisms synchronously. When the body's anaerobic system increases, it metabolizes a compound called pyruvate into lactate (the citric acid cycle). Lactate is then used as another source of energy for short periods.

As the muscles continue to work and your power reserves are insufficient, the acid levels rise (again having nothing to do with lactic acid), and the muscles begin to fail and lose power. Lactate helps to counter the activation of the muscle cells, often felt as tingling or burning when you could no longer maintain running at the same pace. Therefore, as you train your power reserve, lactate levels well above 4 mmol/L are not uncommon. Lactate production is a protective mechanism preventing the body from going too far. When you push yourself too hard, it is not the lactate level that causes you muscle pain. Instead, it is physical damage via micro-tears in the muscle fibrils themselves.

Furthermore, damaged muscles fail to store glycogen optimally. Therefore, it is important to use acceleration-based training using your sensations, which results in better recovery and less muscle injury. The better your body can process lactate, the higher your power reserve, and the ability to vary your pace and run faster.

It is well known that blood lactate reflects the acidosis levels in the muscle (not lactic acid), and this may be a limiting factor in exercise. In our studies, we have not found that the differences in blood lactate correlated with performance. Nevertheless, the higher lactate level in the acceleration group suggests that these mice have better resistance to muscle acidosis than the endurance groups. Indeed, the high intensities achieved during the acceleration training increases the contribution of the anaerobic metabolism for the energy supply. Thus, the mice in the acceleration group may have been accustomed to higher blood lactate levels, suggesting a better tolerance to acidosis, unlike the endurance group being accustomed to low to moderate exercise intensities. Later we will detail workouts that build a tolerance to acidosis.

BIOCHEMISTRY OF LACTATE

Improving your lactate metabolism involves an enzyme called lactate dehydrogenase or LDH for short. This enzyme's job is to change lactate to pyruvate inside the cell—the more LDH you have in the cell, the less muscular fatigue. The exact reasons are not entirely understood. Recall our mouse experiment, where we measured the amount of LDH inside the cells. The enzymatic activity of LDH was higher in the acceleration group's skeletal muscle than the endurance group, leading to greater use of anaerobic metabolism in the acceleration group. This is important because it allows a higher intensity and maintenance of exercise during a marathon (Kaczor 2006). Chronic endurance training has been shown to decrease LDH activity (particularly the muscle isoform, LDH-M) (Bigard 2007). This may explain the differences observed between the acceleration group and the endurance group. From a longevity standpoint, it is well known that the activity of LDH decreases with age. An increase in the activity of LDH through acceleration training may be beneficial in offsetting the decline in anaerobic metabolism with age. In any case, acceleration training is better than LSD endurance training to increase lactate metabolism and LDH activity.

Another enzyme in heart muscle that decreases with age and increases through acceleration training is adenylate kinase (AK). In our study, the enzymatic activity of heart AK was higher in the acceleration group compared to the control group. Its increase in the acceleration group could thus be an additional energy source during intense exercise (Hunter 2004). Concerning the enzymatic activity of creatine kinase (CK), it was higher in skeletal and cardiac muscle of the acceleration group compared to the endurance group. Another example of better energy flow is in the mice who performed the acceleration training allowed them to reach and maintain higher exercise intensities (Tepp 2016).

In research, we have underestimated the declining performance with age, and this has led to more studies on how these crucial enzymes affect energy flux and longevity. These results are consistent with many research studies suggesting that high-intensity training is more efficient than anaerobic endurance training (Tabata 2009). Acceleration training should have a more significant impact than endurance training on anaerobic energy pathways, optimizing our energy flow and resistance to acidosis, leading to better performance in both aged mice and humans.

IT'S NOT ALWAYS ABOUT A HIGH VO2 MAX

We are often taught that an increase in VO2 max is required to increase performance. Remember that VO2 max is not always a sensitive marker of performance because it depends on both cardio-respiratory and metabolic factors in the muscle. Acceleration training affects our aerobic thermal engine (oxidative metabolism). Time and time again, we have shown an increase in mitochondrial respiration, despite not elevating VO2 max. The increase in the number of mitochondria increases the regeneration of PCr and the enzyme citrate synthase (CS). Like LDH and the other enzymes, the enzymatic activity of CS in quadriceps skeletal muscle was higher in the acceleration group compared to the endurance and control groups. This agrees with numerous studies showing a beneficial effect of physical activity on the enzymatic activity of

CS at any age (Malek 2013). This increase in CS activity is commonly related to an increase in mitochondria and an adaptation of aerobic metabolism (Larsen 2012). Moreover, the maximal capacity of mitochondrial respiration (Vmax) (in the presence of ADP) was higher in the gastrocnemius skeletal muscle of the acceleration trained mice compared to the control mice, supplementing the results of CS enzymatic activity. Contrary to our expectations, endurance training did not have the expected effects on the maximum capacity of mitochondrial respiration (Vmax) nor the enzymatic activity of CS, usually impacted by endurance training.

Interestingly, many of these adaptations observed in the acceleration group's skeletal muscle are not visible in the cardiac muscle. This lack of cardiac adaptation in acceleration based training and endurance groups may be due to the short training time (two and four weeks) or the fact that the heart's oxidative capacity was enough to respond to the training stimulus. It has already been reported that CS activity increased in skeletal muscle because of endurance training or HIIT, but not in the heart, suggesting slower response training for cardiac muscle (Siu 2003). For master's athletes, acceleration training is essential since the activity of many of these enzymes decreases with age. Also, mitochondrial dysfunction, especially in the skeletal and heart muscles, significantly impacts older subjects' performance. Acceleration training, which induces better adaptations of aerobic metabolism compared to endurance training, is therefore strongly recommended for the master's level marathoner.

LACTATE AND THE CORI CYCLE

Blood lactate levels depend on the muscle cell production of lactate, its transport outside of the cell (including blood), and its utilization by various organs such as the heart. During exercise, the lactate majority (55 – 70 percent) is re-oxidized by the oxidative (slow) fibers and the heart. However, the lactate can be transported by the arteries of the heart, then transformed into glucose by the liver and the kidneys. Once this happens, this glucose can be used again by the muscles by a process called the Cori cycle, named for the infamous biochemist's Carl and Gerty Cori. Skeletal muscles are the site of significant glycolysis. The heart is a significant consumer of lactate, which is rich in LDH isoenzyme H. Lactate metabolism does not follow a simple linear model. However, it must be realized that lactate formation occurs even in the presence of oxygen since glycolysis is so rapid. The LDH-M enzyme competes with the Krebs cycle, leading to the primary fates of pyruvate being:

1. The oxidation of pyruvate in the tricarboxylic cycle (Krebs cycle)
2. Lactate conversion (LDH reduction)
3. The conversion to alanine (by aminotransferases)

The calculation of power at the maximum steady-state velocity of lactatemia may not truly reflect the lactate's maximum stable state (over time). This is why the www.BillaTraining.com method prefers to underestimate the maximum steady-state velocity of lactate rather than overestimate it by evaluating the lactic threshold by traditional treadmill protocols.

ANTIOXIDANTS AND FREE RADICALS

Another essential aspect of acceleration training is the optimization of antioxidant capabilities. By increasing mitochondrial density and respiration rate in older mice, we can counteract the natural age-related decrease in mitochondria. Acceleration training promotes the antioxidant defense systems of the muscle and other organs. Chronic endurance training may promote higher oxygen consumption in terms of volume and running distance, which accelerates oxidation or promotes "rust" in the muscles. In our study model, just five sessions of acceleration training reduced oxidation by decreasing the number of reactive oxidation species (ROS) produced. Of course, it may take longer to show these benefits in humans but know that acceleration training results in optimizing the antioxidant system.

Cells are generally able to defend against ROS free radical damage using glutathione peroxidase, superoxide dismutase, catalase, and peroxiredoxin dismutase enzymes. Oxygenated chemical species such as free radicals, oxygenated ions, and peroxides, are highly reactive by the presence of oxygen and unmatched electrons. ROS is a chemical species with high reactivity that can damage cells by oxidizing proteins, DNA, and cell membranes. This is one of the current theories of aging, also known as cell senescence or cell death. Interestingly, the concentration of the amino acid taurine was higher in the urine of the acceleration group. Taurine is well known for its antioxidant properties and its ability to reduce the level of free radicals (Shimada 2015). Acceleration training is probably more beneficial than endurance training in increasing oxidative defenses in aged mice and humans.

> ### Increasing Your Lactate Metabolism
>
> Three exercises that can be done to accomplish increasing your lactate metabolism and capacity are (these exercise sessions will be detailed in a later chapter):
>
> - Three-minute repeats. Perform 3-minute repeats at MAS, on 3-minute jog recoveries. This workout is tough, but not demoralizing.
> - 30-30s (version 1). Alternating between 30-second surges at MAS, with 30-second jog recoveries, and doing this for as long as possible. You spend much more time at VO2 max.
> - 30-30s (version 2). This is a very intense session, probably better suited for experienced runners. After a warm-up, hold MAS for 1 minute, which will be about 200 – 400 m. After that fast-paced 1 minute, return to a tempo pace (about 40 percent of MAS), which is about 45 – 60 second/mile slower for 30 seconds. Then you speed back up to 100 percent MAS for 30 seconds and so on. Repeat these 30-30s for as long as you can.

Beyond the metabolic improvements, we must consider progress in terms of performance, which is also the goal beyond the anti-aging benefits. In just five sessions, acceleration training very rapidly increases the maximum running speed reached by the mouse (beyond its MAS). In contrast, endurance training did not affect performance in the first three weeks and decreased in the fourth week of training. This performance decrease could be explained by a loss of efficiency while running at submaximal monotonous racing speeds. It has been shown that training at speeds above MAS (velocity at VO2 max) was necessary to improve VO2 max and performance even for long efforts (MacInnis and Gibala 2017).

CHAPTER 8 SUMMARY

CONCEPT: The benefits of acceleration training exercises are being at MAS and fluctuating blood lactate levels. Anytime you are at MAS, this is where the magic happens, and your body adapts. When we run hard and then slow down, we continue breathing hard for some time afterward. Exercise physiologists used to call this "oxygen debt," but we now know that oxygen has nothing to do with it. As you may recall, our muscles need ATP to break the bonds between actin and myosin in the muscle fibrils and therefore relax the muscle. This "oxygen debt" is a disruption of homeostasis involving ATP regeneration. Restoration of high-energy molecules like ATP and PCr takes only milliseconds in the muscle cells. During these fast-paced recoveries, the body is working to adapt to the excess lactate. This is why the brain, heart, muscles, and diaphragm adapt to using lactate for fuel rather than stealing glucose from your larger hard-working muscles like the quadriceps and gluteus muscles.

APPLICATION: Every endurance athlete is looking for workouts to gain fitness quickly. If you are looking for so-called "magic bullets," lactate training is one place to start. It is important to think of lactate as a friend and not a foe! As discussed earlier, lactate is shuttled from hard working muscles to less hard-working muscles (which are better oxygenated) that can use lactate for energy, thereby sparing the glycolytic pathway or glucose. It is important to train this shuttle in your workouts to use lactate as energy better. The idea is to repeat certain intervals to ramp up your metabolism to something close to VO2 max and hold it there long enough to improve your aerobic capacity. We have found this type of training superior to traditional long intervals.

CHAPTER 9

ENERGY, NUTRITION, AND HUMAN PERFORMANCE

RUNNING A MARATHON IS ALL about energy management. We must manage our energy with our sophisticated hybrid engine. Remember that our hybrid engines use carbohydrates, lipids (fats), and sunlight to produce energy. None of these substances is ever used by the body in isolation, always as a mixture. The combination of the energy substrates used varies with how fast you run, or the intensity of the exercise. With an increase in intensity, a higher percentage of carbohydrates are used, and less fat. From about 85 – 90 percent of the VO2 max, carbohydrates provide the energy for running. PCr and lactate are used as fuel at any intensity. The goal of energy management during a marathon is to use our energy sources efficiently. By starting the marathon quickly, we can take advantage of our fresh legs and abundant fuel sources. By running below our average pace using speed oscillations, we are telling our body to use more fats and to burn lactate efficiently, preserving our glycogen for a fast finish. As we have already amply demonstrated since the first chapter of this book, the marathon is naturally run at a variable speed.

INTEGRATED METABOLISM AND HYBRID ELECTRIC MOTORS

We need to rethink metabolism as an integrated system and no longer in "pathways!" It is a myth that the aerobic system turns off while the anaerobic system turns on. Metabolic energy systems are complex, and we will use many new terms such as ATP, glycolysis, PCr, lactate, lactic acid, alactate (without lactate), fatty acids, and intramuscular triglycerides (lipids). It is useful to compare our bodies to a sophisticated hybrid-electric engine. Even this is undoubtedly an oversimplification, but valuable in understanding how we manage energy during a marathon.

A sophisticated hybrid car engine uses a gasoline-driven internal combustion engine and a battery-powered electric drive system. The batteries are powered by the gasoline engine and produce electricity for later use. In humans, the thermal internal combustion engine is our ability to use glucose and fats for energy in the form of adenosine triphosphate (ATP). We also possess two electric batteries that make ATP: the phospho-creatine system and the anaerobic lactate system. These engine batteries must be interdependent and work together.

Our engines use all the potential electrical and thermal energy synchronously. The electric motor is the anaerobic metabolism, while the gas engine is the aerobic metabolism whose maximum power is the famous VO2 max. These motors are interdependent because we can only mobilize energy at 100 percent of our VO2 max if we simultaneously produce power from our two electric motors. From a physiological standpoint, our pistons (shortening and lengthen our muscle fibers) operate thanks to two electric motors. These two electric motors are battery-powered, a small phosphocreatine high-power battery (anaerobic alactate glycolysis), and a large lactate battery (anaerobic lactate glycolysis). The lactate battery is self-limiting and regulated by the muscular acidity level, again having nothing to with lactic acid. The anaerobic PCr system is the fastest and most powerful and not affected per se by the acidity level. As its name suggests, this system works without oxygen, and does not produce lactate and lasts for about 6 - 15 seconds. The anaerobic lactate system works without oxygen, produces lactate, and lasts for about two minutes.

For over a decade, we have known that these batteries, (anaerobic alactate and lactate) are recharged as soon as the runner lifts his foot. Indeed, PCr is reconstituted by oxygen consumption, and lactate is converted back into pyruvate, which provides energy to the engine. This is the principle of optimal speed variation that will result in faster performance on average than constant speed. Our bodies truly are hybrid vehicles in the diversity of their engines and their operations. The oxygen supply of the combustion engine is delivered by the heart, which distributes in a circuit, which feeds both engines (thermal and electrical) nutrients and oxygen. It also allows for the recycling of metabolites produced by these engines for internal recycling. The only major difference between the human engine and that of a machine is that the electric motor cannot work alone, even during a 100-m sprint! Indeed, the effort of running a 10 second 100-m (elite runners), 30 percent of the energy is provided by the combustible heat engine in the same proportions as a 3000-m effort. A sprinter reaches 100 percent VO2 max from the 3rd second of the race and fights to stay there. Hence the interest for a sprinter like Usain Bolt to possess a high VO2 max. Sprinters too often neglect their aerobic metabolism.

Phosphocreatine and Oxygen Consumption.

Understanding how our energy systems work while running is crucial to understanding why running at variable speeds and listening to your sensations will make you a better marathon runner. ATP production within the oxygen-consuming mitochondria will allow regeneration of PCr at the level of the contractile proteins in proportion to the speed. Varying running speed makes it possible to take advantage of the phosphocreatine-creatine shuttle (PCr/Cr) between the mitochondria and the contractile proteins. Contrary to popular belief, the use of PCr is restricted to a few seconds but occurs throughout exercise through its regeneration by aerobic metabolism.

PCr is degraded to form the ATP required for contractile proteins (PCr + ADP → Cr + ATP) in muscles. Creatine is released in side the cell at the level of the contractile proteins. It then diffuses into the muscle cells' mitochondria, which consume oxygen and produce ATP by a process called mitochondrial respiration. Creatine thus stimulates this production of ATP, allowing the reaction to occur in the opposite direction (Cr + ATP → PCr + ADP). This ATP, newly formed by the mitochondria, is immediately combined with creatine to reform PCr, which will spread to the contractile proteins and allow the reconstitution of PCr stores.

THE IMPORTANCE OF NUTRITION TO INCREASE YOUR SPEED RESERVE

Fueling for a marathon is not just about what you eat during the race but also about how you build metabolic flexibility every day. When and what you eat daily is what becomes important. The conceit that runners can eat anything they want because they burn it off is incredibly old thinking. Nutrition is essential to our health, longevity, performance, healing, and metabolic flexibility. For more than fifty years, researchers have pushed the mantra to consume principally carbohydrates to keep our glycogen stores filled. While carbohydrates are necessary for performance, just not in the way previously thought. Traditionally pasta parties have been held on the *la veille* of the race. Nutritionists, coaches, and researchers have pushed bread, cereal, pasta, highly concentrated gels, bagels, and carbohydrate drinks as anti-bonking survival tools for a marathon. This obsession with carbohydrates in the running world is slowly changing, especially in runners competing in ultra-marathons. We are now finding out that dumping fructose and sugar into our foods increases inflammation, impacts our hormones, and causes insulin resistance. Tim Noakes famously challenged the notion of a high carbohydrate diet after developing type 2 diabetes while having completed over 50 marathons. Metabolic flexibility has always been the key to success in endurance sports. We can store about 1500 – 2000 calories of glycogen in our muscles and about 400 calories of glycogen in our liver. Not many people realize that we have 3000 – 5000 calories of intramuscular TGs available for energy. Finally, we can tap into our immense fat stores under the right conditions.

EXCESS MACRONUTRIENTS CONVERT TO BODY FAT

Many runners follow the mantra of drinking a protein/carbohydrate shake after a training run or race. Replenishing protein, especially in our older athletes, is an excellent thing to do. However, the following will explain why it might not be a good thing to drink your calories! Most athletes consume too many calories following a workout. Excess energy intake from any fuel source can be counterproductive. Any macronutrient can convert to fatty acids and accumulate as excess body fat, typically in the abdominal areas. For example, after a long run, excess dietary carbohydrate primarily fills both liver and muscle glycogen. Glycogen synthesis is complex and takes more than 24 hours to complete. After consuming a recovery drink, the insulin release from the pancreas causes a spike in the hormone insulin, and a thirty-fold increase in glucose transport into the adipocytes. Insulin then initiates the production of glucose into triacylglycerol (TGs) for fat storage in adipocytes. This lipogenic process requires ATP energy as well as B vitamins (biotin, niacin, and pantothenic acid). In the same way, amino acids can be converted to fat.

WHEY PROTEIN – TOO MUCH OF A GOOD THING

Many runners use whey protein after workouts and races. As little children, we were taught the nursery rhyme "Little Miss Muffet Sat on a tuffet/Eating her curds and Whey." For centuries, whey served as animal feed. Early veterinarians noticed how healthy the animals became when fed whey, which led to the research into the benefits of whey protein. In the 1990s, whey protein extraction was perfected and became the purest and most easily absorbed protein source. Today, whey protein is currently marketed as a dietary supplement to facilitate muscular development in response to resistance training. Most athletes do not need whey protein drinks. Save these rich-tasting whey protein drinks for big training days. A good rule of thumb is that any training session under 2 hours does not need to be supplemented. Just eat a real whole food meal, and be sure to sit down and enjoy it in the French way! Eat real food and experiment to see what works for you.

Olympic Runner Brenda Martinez

Brenda Martinez is an American Olympic track and field athlete, specializing in middle distance races. She won a silver medal in the 800-m at the IAAF World Championships. Brenda's journey into utilizing a lower carbohydrate approach is an excellent example. In her early twenties, weight was never an issue. She was able to maintain a weight below 120 lbs eating a predominantly high carbohydrate diet. She set world records and made the USA Olympic team. Into her thirties, she found that maintaining her weight was not so straightforward. She was unable to decrease her weight healthily, below 127 lbs. Family history, lab, and genetic tests showed that Brenda had a propensity for insulin resistance, especially given her Latino heritage. Experimenting with various types of diets, and even vegetarian for a short period, nothing seemed to help her get down to her competitive weight in a healthy manner. She sustained several injuries during this period of her life. Finally, she decided to limit her carbohydrates to about 100 grams a day and integrating fasted

> training runs. Within months, her weight dropped to 120 lbs., injury-free, and runs PRs into her thirties. She cut out the glucose/carbohydrate drinks after workouts and is now using carbohydrates more strategically. As she increases the frequency of her anaerobic workouts, she will increase the number of carbohydrates and proteins in her workouts. In Brenda's case, the periodization of carbohydrates, according to her physiology, has been a success. Brenda is planning on competing in the 2021 Olympic games in Japan (International Olympic Committee decided to move the games due to the COVID-19 virus).

FATS ARE IMPORTANT

We use fats every day of our lives. Every night when you sleep, for example, fats are being used as energy, and our metabolism goes into something called ketosis. Lipid and carbohydrate metabolism are always simultaneously, and we cannot survive otherwise. The degree of lipid metabolism is what is in play. Glucose is the metabolic bully that cuts to the front of the energy partitioning line. This is what keeps us from using fats for energy efficiently. Thus, the concept of optimizing your fat metabolism. We have been conditioned to think that we burn either fat or carbohydrates. Nothing could be farther from the truth, fats and carbohydrates burn synchronously, just like our hybrid engines. We all burn fats and carbohydrates differently. Even a lean individual has a reserve of 60,000 – 100,000 fat calories available as energy.

When we use fat for energy, it is virtually endless. When fat is used as energy, TGs are broken down into glycerol and fatty acid components. Blood transports the free fatty acids released from adipocytes and bound to a protein called plasma albumin. The fatty acids are taken up by the cell, go into the mitochondria, and make ATP through a complicated process called beta-oxidation. People often confuse beta-oxidation for ketosis; they are separate things. The fatty acids are converted into a molecule called acetyl-CoA and then enters the citric acid cycle (CAC) to generate ATP. Recall that acetyl-CoA enters the CAC by combining with oxaloacetate to form citrate.

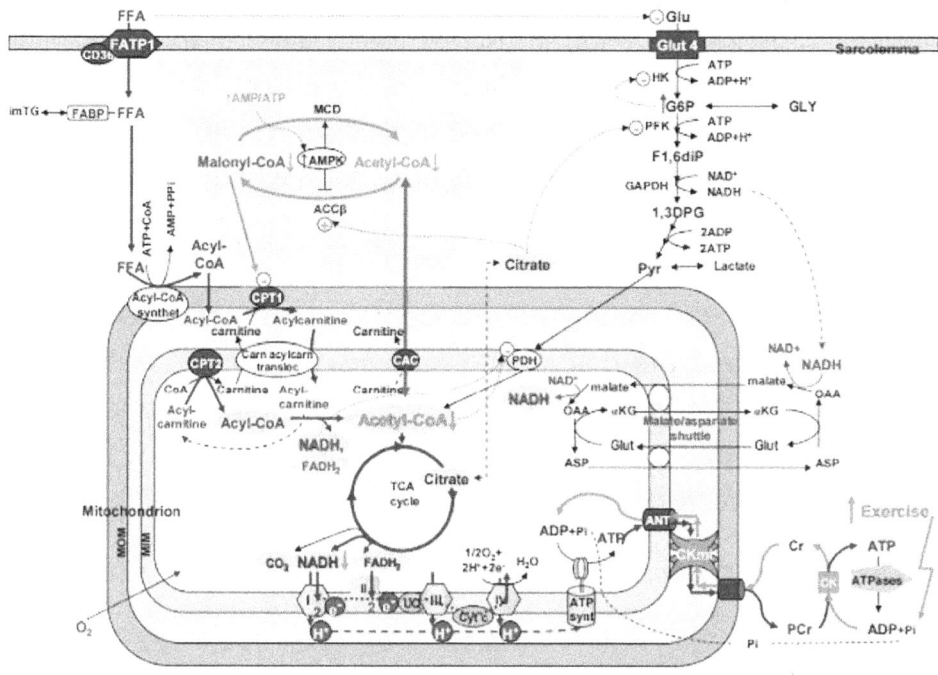

Figure 24. Citric acid cycle. The metabolic processes for making energy from glucose and fat inside of the mitochondria.

Ketones and energy

The word ketone, ketosis, nutritional ketosis, ketogenic diet are all big buzzwords. We often hear the recommendation to try a low carb diet or a ketogenic diet. While there's merit to these approaches, it is important to remember that we are deriving most of our energy from lipids. Ketones are used as energy, but they are a sideshow compared to using fatty acids. Ketones are produced when we severely restrict carbohydrates and principally made in the liver from the same acetyl-CoA that enters the CAC. We don't know a lot about this phenomenon because ketones are used so quickly; we cannot measure this effect. In principle, ketone's primary use is as an energy source for the brain to prevent neural fatigue. Ketones are also involved in controlling inflammation, longevity, intestinal cell health, and much more. Test your blood or urine ketones after a long run; they are often elevated.

Lipid metabolism increases during exercise for several reasons: a low carbohydrate state, fasting, or prolonged physical activity. An excellent example of this is how our leg muscles utilize intramuscular TGs for energy. Intramuscular TGs are fascinating. They can provide us with more than 3000 calories of energy at any given time. Recall that muscle glycogen can provide about 2000 calories, but it is easier to utilize. Intramuscular TGs provide us with much of the energy needed to run a marathon. Energy releases within the muscle fibers when TGs are broken down via hormones called HSL (hormone-sensitive lipase). The various lipid mobilizing hormones are epinephrine, norepinephrine, glucagon, and growth hormone. Note that lactate, ketones, and insulin all inhibit fatty acid mobilization and lipid use for energy. Intracellular and extracellular lipid molecules usually supply between 30 – 80 percent of the energy for exercise, depending on three factors:

- Individual nutrition status
- Insulin sensitivity
- Physical fitness level

INTENSITY AND DURATION OF PHYSICAL ACTIVITY

Fats serve as the primary energy fuel during running, especially when intense, long-duration activity depletes glycogen. Furthermore, enzymatic adaptations enhance lipid oxidation capacity with prolonged exposure to a higher-fat, low-carbohydrate diet during physical activity. Interestingly, fatty acid breakdown depends on in part on a continual background level of carbohydrate breakdown. This is why you might have heard that "fats burn in the flame of a carbohydrate drip." The energy released from lipids is indeed slower than the energy released from carbohydrates. Aerobic training certainly enhances the energy generated by lipid breakdown, but it is still about half of the value achieved from carbohydrates. This explains why glycogen depletion decreases our ability to sustain a certain pace, especially in lesser trained individuals. Low sugar or hypoglycemic conditions coincide with "central" or neural fatigue. One thing you can do to make your marathon more enjoyable from an energy standpoint is to optimize your fat metabolism and strategically consume carbohydrates.

Optimizing your fat metabolism (OFM) often invokes some difficult choices. The average marathon runner will need to cut down on carbohydrate consumption. Eating things like pasta, cereals, bread, and even fruits will impede your fat optimization. You will need to practice things like running fasted and time restrict eating. Undoubtedly, moving away from drinking your calories is a good start. You may see some runners, usually elite, who can consume large amounts of carbohydrates and stay very fit and run fast. Realize those elite runners train several hours per day, and their metabolisms are already optimized to burn fat. Of course, there are differences between elite runners, but they all can use fats and glucose better than the average runner. Most runners overconsume carbohydrates. It is the average runner wanting to complete a marathon that will benefit the most by optimizing their fat metabolism. Take a chance and educate yourself on how to live an OFM lifestyle. You will see that it is remarkably similar to a traditional French lifestyle!

LIPOX-MAX THEORY – RUNNING TO BURN FAT

As François Péronnet (French-Canadian exercise physiologist) correctly states – "The theory of lipox-max is very clear, but in practice, it becomes much less so."

Who doesn't want to burn more fat? The lure of burning fat and losing weight attracts many runners to the sport. It was a popular theory in exercise physiology to find the speed or pace that would burn the most fat for energy. It was thought that if we wish to oxidize the largest amount of lipids possible during exercise, we must run at lower intensities. The optimal intensity to oxidize lipids must be high enough to allow a significant energy expenditure, but not too much, as to avoid using too much carbohydrate. We can also address another physiological concept of the 1990s currently used by some runners wanting to lose weight. This is the pace that gives the highest fat or lipid oxidation (in grams per minute): the lipox-max.

The top of the curve in Figure 25 is the intensity at which the lipid oxidation rate peaks. This intensity, called fat-max or lipox-max, is simple to determine during an exercise by measuring the volume and composition of exhaled gases. We calculate the energy expenditure, and we establish the relative share of energy expended from the oxidation of carbohydrates and that of lipids. This calculation is made from the respiratory quotient or RQ, which is the ratio between the expired volume of carbon dioxide (CO_2) and the volume of oxygen (O2) consumed. (RQ = VCO2/VO2). The RQ associated with carbohydrate oxidation is 1.0, and that associated with lipid oxidation is approximately 0.7. A RQ of about 0.85 (halfway between the two extremes) indicates that half of the energy is provided by the oxidation of carbohydrates and the other half by the oxidation of lipids. Thus, by combining the RQ information with the measure of energy expenditure, we can calculate the intensity of the exercise that corresponds to the maximum rate of lipid oxidation. In adults, lipox-max varies from about 30 – 75 percent of VO2 max.

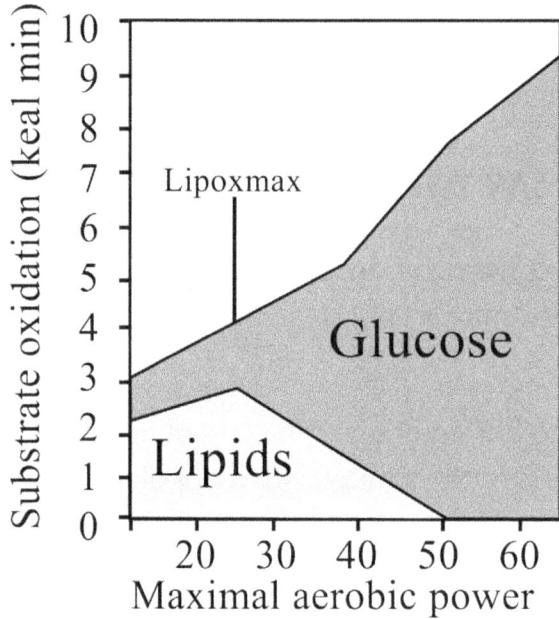

Figure 25. Relationship between substrate oxidation (carbohydrates/lipids) and maximum aerobic power (MAP).

Here are the problems with the lipox-max theory

1. The lipox-max is not a peak, nor is it a precise point. The lipid consumption curve peak is a single "bump," whereas the maximum rate of lipid oxidation exists in a wide range of intensities. One study tested cyclists of all levels and found that the lipox-max corresponded to an exercise intensity of 64 percent of VO2 max. But the lipox-max zone ranged from 55 – 72 percent of VO2 max, that is, at intensities corresponding to the lipox-max zone for most of the population.

2. The lipox-max continuously changes. The lipox-max is not an immutable characteristic of the runner. It varies according to the level of form and especially the diet. Indeed, our sport organizes its carbohydrate formula according to the energy contributions. This results in a marked increase in the RQ for those who perform exercise following a high carbohydrate diet.

3. The oxidation of the lipids continues well after an effort is finished!

4. The lipox max can be greatly increased by eating a higher fat, lower carbohydrate diet, independent of exercise.

5. Lipox-max training is not effective.

In summary, the energetics and nutrition for the marathon runner is complex and often debated. It is important to find what works for you and be open to trying new things. There are differences in the nutrition of an elite versus an amateur runner. We find that most runners overconsume carbohydrates. Recognize that fats, carbohydrates, and protein are essential for the marathon runner.

CHAPTER 9 SUMMARY

CONCEPT: Running a marathon is all about energy management. Understanding how our energy systems work while running is crucial to understanding why running at variable speeds and listening to your sensations will make you a better marathon runner. ATP production within the oxygen-consuming mitochondria will allow regeneration of PCr at the level of the contractile proteins in proportion to the speed. Varying running speed makes it possible to take advantage of the phosphocreatine-creatine shuttle (PCr/Cr) between the mitochondria and the contractile proteins. Contrary to popular belief, the use of PCr is not restricted to a few seconds but occurs throughout exercise through its regeneration by aerobic metabolism.

APPLICATION: By running below our average pace using speed oscillations, we tell our body to use more fats and to burn lactate efficiently, preserving our carbohydrates for a fast finish. As we have already amply demonstrated since the first chapter of this book, the marathon is naturally run at a variable speed.

We must manage our energy with our complex hybrid engine. Remember that our hybrid engines use carbohydrates, lipids (fats), and sunlight to produce energy. None of these substances is ever used by the body in isolation, always as a mixture. The combination of the energy substrates used varies with how fast you run, or the intensity of the exercise. As exercise intensity increases, a higher percentage of carbohydrates are used, and less fat. From about 85 – 90 percent of the VO2 max, carbohydrates provide the energy for running. PCr and lactate are used as fuel at any intensity. The goal of energy management during a marathon is to use our energy sources efficiently. By starting the marathon quickly, we can take advantage of our fresh legs and abundant fuel sources.

CHAPTER 10

RELATIONSHIP BETWEEN SPEED, VO2 MAX, MAS AND PERFORMANCE

THE WORLD'S BEST RUNNERS POSSESS a high VO2 max and superior running economy, which allows a remarkably high capacity to consume oxygen during intense levels of running. While VO2 max is an excellent predictor of performance, its correlation to athletic success is only 20 – 40 percent. For example, there are many marathon winners with relatively low VO2 max scores. Many other factors, such as sustainable lactate threshold, motivation, environment, neural fatigue, and economy, play important roles in marathon success. It is true that the higher VO2 max, the higher the potential for athletic success. In the general population, VO2 max is about 45-50 ml/kg/min in men; 57 in US college track male athletes, and this number declines to less than 35 in the elderly. The highest VO2 max scores recorded were in Norwegian athletes, Bjorn Dahlie, a male cross-country skier (94 ml/kg/min), and Oskar Svendsen, a professional cyclist (97.5 ml/kg/min). A problem with VO2 max is that it is sport dependent, and the administration of these tests is highly variable. A VO2 max measured in a cyclist cannot be construed that they will have an equivocal VO2 max while running or rowing. Body mass significantly affects VO2 max, a runner with a low body mass will have a higher VO2 max than a runner with a high body mass. Aside from sports, VO2 max importantly predicts overall health and mortality. A higher VO2 max is associated with longer lifespan, higher quality of life, reduced risk of cardiovascular disease and stroke, diabetes, cancer, and even reduce the risk of suicide and depression. It is interesting to compare a human's VO2 max with other animals. We do not fare so well as many other mammals consume oxygen at much faster rates. A humans' VO2 max is equivalent to that of a rat or pig. Thus, the reason rats are often used in studies of VO2 max. Humans have about half the VO2 max as horses and dogs. The VO2 max of a hummingbird is about 600 ml/kg/min.

ENERGY COST OF RUNNING

When you watch a good runner, that person has optimized their energy cost of running. Knowing your energy cost and economy of running is essential. By far, the most significant gains in running times are made by optimizing your running economy. The energy that goes into running affects every aspect of physiology, mechanics, and the environment. Whether running or walking, the energy is about the same; the primary difference being that energy is used faster at higher speeds. The energy cost of running is higher for smaller humans and animals. Running involves little work against the environment, and rather the work is done by muscles, ligaments, and tendons lifting and accelerating the extremities. The VO2 max of the quadriceps is higher when they are isolated in sports like running or cycling than whole-body exercises. Regardless of the amount of work done by the muscles, they must activate and develop the force necessary to support the limbs' weight. This is what we refer to as the energy cost and the economy of running.

The energy cost of running (CE) has been traditionally quantified from mass-specific oxygen uptake. Relatively little is known about the potpourri of physiological, environmental, structural, and mechanical factors that affect the aerobic demands of running. Factors like tendon stiffness, foot strike, ankle mobility, skeletal muscle contraction, muscle fibril type, high or low altitude, force-velocity relationship of the muscles, temperature, hydration, footwear, running surface, calf thickness, stride frequency, pacers, and the list continues. Elite runners consider all these factors to optimize their running performance by even one percent; this is known as the science of marginal gains. Taking advantage of these marginal gains were instrumental for Kipchoge to break the 2-hour marathon. It is thought that his specialized carbon plated shoes may have given him a one percent gain to his running economy. These seemingly small improvements often account for the breakthroughs witnessed in elite and amateur running athletes.

A better running economy equates to more efficiently using oxygen. Morgan (1989) noted that the running economy is defined as the steady-state VO2 for given running speed, and he determined how to calculate VO2 max during a progressively increasing treadmill exercise. Most runners reach this steady-state in about three minutes, and trained individuals reach steady-state faster than those who are less fit. It is also important to note the differences in running on a treadmill vs. running outside: a treadmill significantly underestimates the energy cost of running.

> ### The History of the Treadmill
>
> Exercising on a treadmill seems like torture, and this is no coincidence! In the 1800s the English developed a machine called the "tread-wheel" to reform convicts. Prisoners were forced to step on the twenty-four spokes of a large paddle wheel, resembling the modern Stairmaster®. The paddle wheel functioned to crush grain, hence the name "treadmill." The exertion, in combination with inadequate nutrition, led to injuries and exhaustion, and even death. In England, the treadmill persisted until the late nineteenth century, abandoned because it was considered cruel and unusual punishment. In the 1960s, the famous Dr. Cooper demonstrated the health benefits of aerobic exercise, and the treadmill made a triumphant return. Today, well-paid personal trainers have taken prison guards' place as we continue the use of treadmills! Yes, exercise treadmills have their advantages, but we feel the disadvantages outweigh the advantages. Runners develop weak running economy such as a bouncy gait and monotonous pace. Learn to run outside as nature intended!

HOW MAS AND VO2 MAX RELATES TO THE ENERGY COST OF RUNNING

In academics, we use vVO2 max instead of MAS. vVO2 max can be calculated from VO2 max measurements and the CE. We will show you how to measure MAS yourself. Note that different scientific papers use different symbols, such as Cr to denote the energy cost of running. Here we will use CE. And don't worry if you are unable to follow the equations, it is just for illustrating the principles of the energy cost of running. Morgan tested runners who completed a 5-minute run at 12.8 km/hr during three different sessions followed by four 6-minute runs at 13.8, 14.9, 16.1, and 17.6 km/hr respectively, with five minutes of recovery between each session. The relation between VO2 and velocity was then plotted, and vVO2 max (MAS) was estimated by extrapolation from the known value of VO2 max (figure 26).

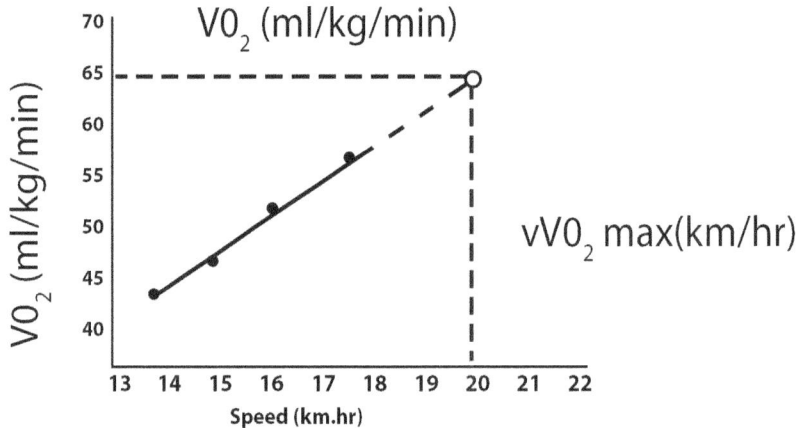

Figure 26. The relation between travel speeds and oxygen consumed. The regression line is calculated (solid line) using the values obtained for under maximal travel speeds (solid circles). The vVO2 max value is then obtained by extending this line (dotted line) to the known value of the VO2 max (hollow circle).

The metabolic power (E) necessary to move at speed (v) is equal to the product of this same speed by the energy cost of the running (CE):

$$E = CE \times V$$

Under maximal conditions, the equation becomes:

$$V\,max = E\,max/CE$$

Finally, under maximal aerobic conditions, since E depends essentially on VO2 max, we obtain the following equation:

$$V\ max = (F \times VO2\ max)/CE$$

where V end is the speed of endurance, and F is the maximum fraction of VO2 max that can be maintained over the exercise duration. For F equal to 1, we can then determine Vmax (maximum velocity) equal to:

$$Vmax = VO2\ max/CE$$

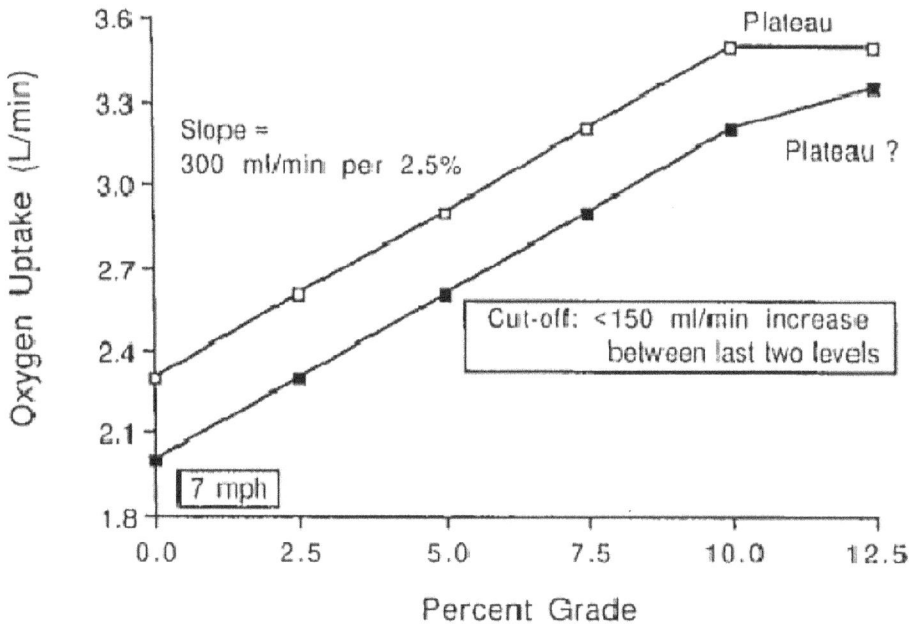

Figure 27. Kinetics of VO2 during an incremental test of two representative subjects, both of which validated secondary criteria for VO2 max. One of them (white square) shows a plateau of VO2 max. Conversely, the second (black square) does not show a plateau of VO2 max (Howley 1995).

VO2 MAX – IS THE CEILING FLAT?

In many books and Internet running blogs, the ceiling of VO2 max is thought to be flat beyond a certain point. This is not entirely the case. It is accepted that a ceiling of VO2 max must be observed (figure 27) despite an increase in the speed and power of the exercise. We thus reach a linear relationship between power, speed, and oxygen consumption. The value of the slope of this linear relation is 3.5 (ml/kg/min each km/hr), a well-known value used by "Internet gurus" who adore the estimation of their VO2 max from MAS or vVO2 max. We, therefore, expect a magnificent plateau of VO2 max. Nevertheless, this is not always the case.

In real life, we assume that the slope of the equation VO2/velocity is **on average** is equal to 3.5 ml/kg/min each time the runner increases his speed by 1 km/hr. The slope of the relation VO2/speed is characteristic of an individual's running economy, ranging from 3 – 4 ml of O2/kg/km/hr. Note that this variance is large, and therefore, it is an audacious claim to estimate VO2 max by simply multiplying the peak speed of the VAMEVAL test by 3.5 (often done on the Internet running blogs). In addition, the peak speed attained is not systematically the lowest speed that solicits VO2 max in a VAMEVAL test. Even worse, this test does not account for reaching VO2 max over time for speeds just above the critical speed (the maximum steady-state velocity of blood lactate). Polish physiologist Jerzy Zoladz, who was an 800-m runner, highlighted the non-linearity of the VO2/velocity relationship. He observed an inflection of actual VO2 max from what was expected. The critical finding is that the energy cost of increasing the running speed was not constant, as was previously thought. In 2010, Dr. Billat's research demonstrated that by varying the speed (or power) at the end of a VAMEVAL test, VO2 increases beyond the obtained VO2 max. As a runner increases speed, VO2 continues to increase or remains at the plateau at VO2 max. What this means for you is that you may be pushing yourself too hard during your intervals. Optimal training programs start with optimal training numbers. Many coaches push their runners to hold a constant speed during an interval, resulting in less time spent at VO2 max. Everything is in the dosage of the decline and the rise of speed. It is this "discovery" that has put us on the path of optimal speed variation! Simply said, "learn to slow down, and you will go faster."

> ## Running a Sub 2 hour and 30 marathon at age 60
>
> Fifty-nine-year-old Irishman Tommy Hughes has a VO2 max of 65.4 ml/kg/min, remarkable for his age. It is nearly double that for a normal man

> his age. He also holds the world record for the fastest marathon in his age group at two hours, twenty-seven minutes, and 52 seconds. He's running the marathon at 90 percent of his VO2 max (which is entirely another discussion). Hughes running economy is said to be incredible, and he still trains just about every day. He notes that speed decreases with age, but if you just keep running, you can improve your marathon times. Hughes' example supports that by continuing training hard into our later years, VO2 max can be increased. The trick is to stay healthy because an injury will put you out for six months. As a side note, it is relatively easier for a master's athlete to run at a higher VO2 because of lower muscle mass, lower max heart rate, and higher thresholds relative to their VO2 max.

A DEEPER LOOK INTO USING MAS AS A TRAINING TOOL – T LIMIT

Measuring MAS and VO2 max in the field is invaluable to understand. Knowing your velocity where you touch VO2 max is essential in developing a minimalistic acceleration-based training program. For this, we use a value called the T limit (T-lim), which is defined as the time a runner can maintain MAS. T-lim is measured by having the runner push until exhaustion at MAS, and the time recorded is T-lim. We know that the velocity reached VO2 max is called MAS, keep in mind this is not sprint speed. However, in addition to the running speed, it is necessary to set the exercises' duration. **An exercise can only be correctly defined if we know the pace at which it is performed and its duration.** Only by knowing how fast you run at VO2 max and how long you can run at this speed can you improve your running quickly. While 3 – 6 percent may not seem like much, in elite runners, this represents a considerable improvement. The gains will be even higher in non-elite runners.

Knowing these speeds takes the guesswork out of your training. MAS has shown to be highly predictive of endurance exercise performance and training program design. MAS explains why a runner with a lower VO2 max can perform better than another athlete with a higher VO2 max. Again, MAS is defined as the minimum speed at which the maximal oxygen consumption (VO2 max) occurs. Elite or amateur, knowing your T-lim can be important in devising a successful marathon training program. T-lim is a measurement of "truth," where a runner's true abilities lie. For intervals to work, you must have strong reference points around which to structure workouts. These reference points are MAS and T-lim.

Take the example of the following runner, their speed at MAS is 5 m/s, but their max sprint speed is 10 m/s. What we want to know is the T-lim at 5 m/s, not max sprint speed. Our lab studied T-lim at various percentages of the MAS. We did this because there is a lot of individual variability in measuring the T-lim. The errors made while measuring the MAS are magnified when the T-lim is measured. We found that most adults can hold T-lim between 3 - 9 minutes. Based on this observation, Dr. Billat proposed a new definition of MAS, or rather a new concept: the velocity allowing one to solicit VO2 max for as long as possible.

We can thus suppose that this speed, which would make it possible to maximally solicit the oxygen transport system, for as long as possible, is preferred if the objective of the training is the improvement of VO2 max. At BillaTraining.com, we design workouts to keep you close to VO2 max, but at your own pace. This concept applies to both amateur and elite runners alike. The point of all of this is how sports physiologists were mistaken for so many years because we thought that training at constant speed was the key to effective training. It is time to break free from the paradigm of constant speeds and time limits. These two paradigms in training lead to only one result - the catastrophe of terminal fatigue (cracking) during the race without catching up before terminal fatigue arises. Fatigue is defined as the impossibility of sustaining a given power or speed. We can then begin to dream of disappearance of this notion of fatigue since we do not seek the maintenance of constant speed. The marathon is a series of speed choices and decision making that simultaneously reminds us of what it is to live by running free.

TESTING MAS IN REAL-WORLD CONDITIONS

MAS has brought a lot of attention to the running world in the last twenty years. To simulate real-world conditions, Dr. Billat measured the lowest speed at VO2 max to perform these calculations under actual conditions used by athletes during training and racing. You will learn that testing MAS in the field liberates you from the treadmill and is easier to perform than traditional VO2 max testing. At BillaTraining.com, our goal is for you to look forward to testing MAS versus dreading a VO2 max test. We believe that the field test is preferable if the subject is evaluated for training purposes. There are many methods to assess MAS but realize values obtained for MAS are not the same on an outdoor track compared to a treadmill. The differences in speed can be attributed to aerodynamic factors that do not exist on the treadmill. If using a treadmill, set the slope to 1 percent, because the differences in speed are negligible near-maximum speeds. In these studies, the incline of the treadmill is intended to impose a resistance meant to be a substitute for the conditions of the field tests.

PROTOCOLS FOR MEASURING THE SPEED AT MAS IN THE LABORATORY

In the laboratory, MAS is normally assessed using an incremental treadmill test over 5 or 6 minutes while measuring the oxygen consumption over several incremental stages until the point at which oxygen consumption does not increase further. The speed or velocity at which this point occurs is the runner's MAS. Most training protocols are designed from inside a laboratory using a treadmill that involves incremental intensities. For trained subjects, the treadmill test (no slope) starts at 12 km/hr. The speed of the treadmill is then increased from 2 km/hr every three minutes up to 80 percent of the fastest speed of the subjects over 3000-m. The speed increases are then set to 1 km/hr. The lowest speed for which the VO2 max is reached is recorded, which is the MAS.

HOW TO MEASURE YOUR OWN MAS AND T-LIM IN THE FIELD

At BillaTraining.com, we construct a training regime based on the individual. Measuring MAS can be done using the UMTT, Cooper, or RABIT tests. These tests are best done on a track with little wind or on a treadmill. We prefer to do these tests in the field—warm-up at an easy pace for about 15 to 30 minutes. The goal of any MAS test is to have a simple, repeatable, and fast measurement of the MAS.

University of Montreal Track Test – UMTT

University of Montreal physiologists Léger and Boucher (1980) were the first to propose an indirect, progressive, continuous, and maximal speed test initially used to evaluate the VO2 max of the subjects. The University of Montreal Run Track Test (UMTT), begins at a speed of 6 km/hr (3.7 mph), which is about 5 METs. A MET stands for Metabolic Equivalent Table, where 1 MET represents the oxygen consumption at rest, i.e., 3.5 ml/kg/min. The velocity is then increased by 1.2 km/hr (1 MET) in 2-minute increments. The test ends when the subject is no longer able to keep pace with the imposed pace. The authors have denoted this speed as vUMTT. For calculation purposes, it is easier to perform the test using km/hr.

Equipment Required: 400-meter running track, marker cones, measuring tape, audio tones.

Procedure: A level 400 meter running track, marker cones are placed every 50 meters along the track. The first stage is set at a walking speed of 6 km/hr, which is 5 METS. The speed is then increased to 1.2 km per hour (1 MET) every 2 minutes. The change in speed in indicated by pre-recorded audio cues. Use a preset timer that beeps or have someone call out the change in speeds. The test is stopped when the runners fall five or more meters short of the designated marker, or when the runner feels they cannot continue.

Scoring: The score is the distance covered in meters, multiply by 12, and the runner has his/her MAS.

The following equation can be used to convert the score into VO2 max.

$$VO2max = 1.353 + (3.163 \times \text{speed of last stage}) + ((0.0122586 \times (\text{speed of last stage}))$$

Target population: This test is suitable for team sports such as football, basketball, baseball, etc.

Advantages: The test is relatively easy to perform, and large groups can perform the test at the same time.

Disadvantages: This is a maximal test that requires a reasonable level of fitness. Thus, prescribing this test to sedentary individuals may not be applicable. The test is conducted outdoors. Thus environmental conditions can affect the test. Practice and motivation levels also influence the score attained.

Cooper Test

This test consists of a 12-minute maximal run in which runner attempt to cover as much distance as possible in 12 minutes.

Equipment required: A flat running track, marker cones, recording sheets, and a stopwatch.

Procedure: Place markers at set intervals around the track to aid in measuring the completed distance. Or use a GPS running watch. The athletes run for 12 minutes, and the total distance covered is recorded. Walking is permitted, but each runner is encouraged to cover as much distance as possible in the 12 minutes.

Scoring: Several equations can be used to calculate VO2 max from the distance score. There are also Cooper test norm tables that can be utilized.

$$VO2\ max = (35.97 \times miles) - 11.29$$

$$VO2\ max = (22.35 \times kilometers) - 11.29$$

Advantages: The Cooper test can be used for most populations, including school children. Large groups can be tested at once outdoors. The test can be done on a treadmill. It is a simple and inexpensive test to perform.

Disadvantages: The reliability of this test depends on practice, pacing strategies, and the runner's motivation level.

(See chart on next page.)

Age		Very good	Good	Average	Bad	Very bad
13-14	M	2700+ m	2400 - 2700 m	2200 - 2399 m	2100 - 2199 m	2100- m
	F	2000+ m	1900 - 2000 m	1600 - 1899 m	1500 - 1599 m	1500- m
15-16	M	2800+ m	2500 - 2800 m	2300 - 2499 m	2200 - 2299 m	2200- m
	F	2100+ m	2000 - 2100 m	1700 - 1999 m	1600 - 1699 m	1600- m
17-20	M	3000+ m	2700 - 3000 m	2500 - 2699 m	2300 - 2499 m	2300- m
	F	2300+ m	2100 - 2300 m	1800 - 2099 m	1700 - 1799 m	1700- m
20-29	M	2800+ m	2400 - 2800 m	2200 - 2399 m	1600 - 2199 m	1600- m
	F	2700+ m	2200 - 2700 m	1800 - 2199 m	1500 - 1799 m	1500- m
30-39	M	2700+ m	2300 - 2700 m	1900 - 2299 m	1500 - 1899 m	1500- m
	F	2500+ m	2000 - 2500 m	1700 - 1999 m	1400 - 1699 m	1400- m
40-49	M	2500+ m	2100 - 2500 m	1700 - 2099 m	1400 - 1699 m	1400- m
	F	2300+ m	1900 - 2300 m	1500 - 1899 m	1200 - 1499 m	1200- m
50+	M	2400+ m	2000 - 2400 m	1600 - 1999 m	1300 - 1599 m	1300- m
	F	2200+ m	1700 - 2200 m	1400 - 1699 m	1100 - 1399 m	1100- m

Figure 28. Cooper Test Chart

RABIT test

At BillaTraining.com, we developed the RABIT test to measure MAS and VO2 max in the field. The RABIT test is performed using a GPS equipped running watch. Be sure that you are well-rested. After a proper warm-up, follow the protocol according to your sensations: walking pace, easy pace, moderate pace, hard pace, and sprint pace.

- Easy pace for 10 minutes, followed by 1-minute walking pace
- Sprint for 10 seconds, followed by 1-minute walking pace

- Medium pace for 5 minutes, followed by 1-minute walking pace

- Hard pace for 3 minutes, followed by 1-minute walking pace

- Sprint for 30 seconds, followed by a 1-minute walking pace

- Easy pace for 10 minutes, and the test is done

Download the activity in the application, (usually Polar or Garmin), send the TCX or GPX file to BillaTraining.com and we will give the MAS and estimated VO2 max for that activity.

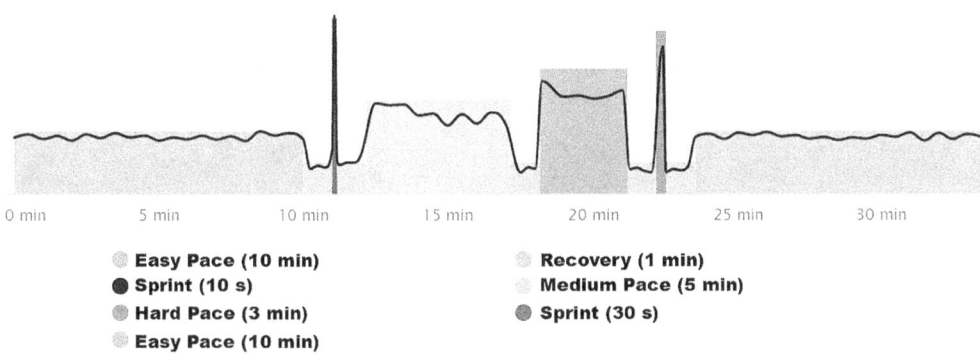

Figure 29. The RABIT test by BillaTraining.com

CHAPTER 10 SUMMARY

CONCEPT: Relationship between Speed at VO2 max, MAS, and Performance. The world's best runners possess a high VO2 max and superior running economy, which allows a remarkably high capacity to consume oxygen during intense levels of running. While VO2 max is an excellent predictor of performance, its correlation to athletic success is only 20 to 40 percent. For example, there are many marathon winners with relatively low VO2 max scores. Many other factors such as sustainable lactate threshold, motivation, environment, neural fatigue, and economy play important roles in marathon success. When you watch a good runner, that person has optimized their energy cost of running. Knowing your energy cost and economy of running is important. By far, the most significant gains in running times are done by optimizing your running economy. The energy that goes into running affects every aspect of physiology, mechanics, and the environment.

APPLICATION: How to measure your own MAS and T-lim. At BillaTraining.com, we construct a training plan based on the individual. Measuring MAS can be done using the UMTT, Cooper, or RABIT tests. These tests are best done on a track with little wind or on a treadmill. We prefer to do these tests in the field and warm up at an easy pace for about 15 to 30 minutes. Given that there are many methods for testing MAS, testing MAS for your workout programs is important. The goal of any MAS test is to have a simple, repeatable, and fast measurement of the MAS.

CHAPTER 11

CRITICAL SPEED CONCEPT

Let's take a closer look at aerobic speeds and the concept of critical speed. Critical speed (CS) is defined as the race pace for any endurance event lasting between 30 and 60 minutes. It also applies to marathon running and other distances. Critical speed is different from MAS. Recall that MAS is the slowest speed from which VO2 max is plateaued. But applying MAS to a long endurance race, such as a marathon, is not applicable in the real-world. This is why the CS concept was developed and is helpful in a marathon if you want to race to your full potential. CS is an important tool in predicting marathon performance, and the runner with the fastest critical speed should theoretically win the race. Critical speed is easy to perform and is an important tool in determining fitness level and predicting performance. Using CS is a tool advanced coaches use to guide athletes to keep their easy days easy and hard days hard. Determining your CS is much easier than determining your anaerobic or lactate threshold, and no expensive equipment is needed. An approximation of CS can be determined by running 10 – 15 percent below MAS for 3 – 5 minutes to reach the reference VO2 max on a treadmill. This speed, beyond which it is no longer possible to remain at a stable VO2 without drifting to VO2 max, is called the "critical speed." The CS concept was developed as a power associated with VO2 max (maximum aerobic power).

The Concept of CS in Research

For the more curious among you, perhaps exercise physiologists or master's students, CS is important in research. The critical speed is deduced from the relationship between time to exhaustion (T-lim) and the distance (D-lim). Recall that T-lim is found by running at constant velocity (MAS) until exhaustion. Critical speed is described by a linear relationship using the equation Dlim = a = b x tlim. It is the slope of the line expressing the evolution of the time limit (T-lim) according to the limit distance (D lim). The graph below shows a runner's personal best over 1500 and 5000-m. The slope is close to the speed at which the lactate level of the runner reaches 4 mmol/L and represents the maximum speed or power representing a stable state of lactate in the blood (Lechevalier 1989). Said in another way, the loss of speed over 1500 – 5000-m is linear for the same runner. This corresponds to the solicitation of the aerobic metabolism with prolonging the distance.

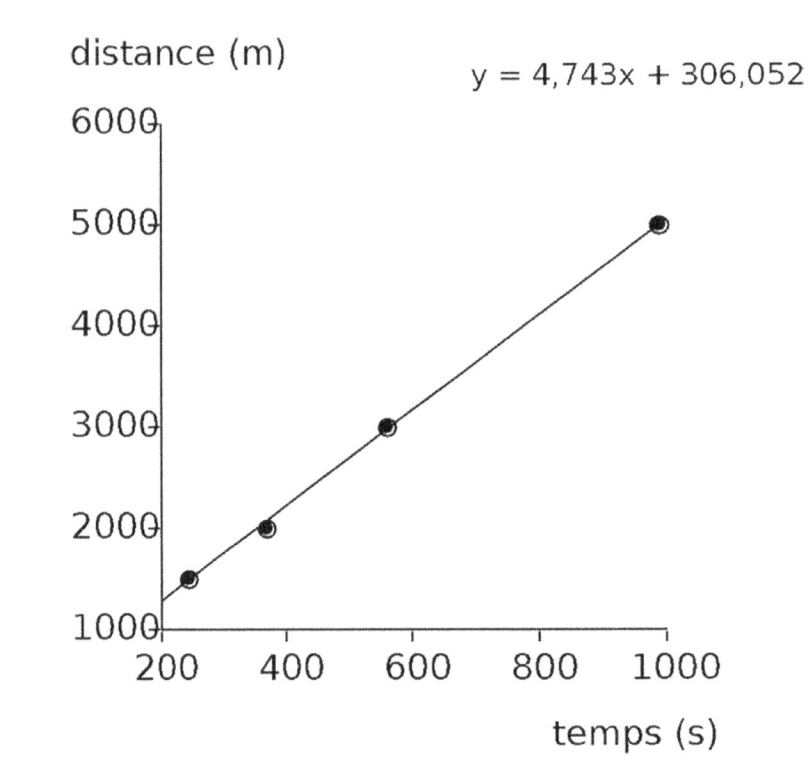

Figure 30. The relation between time and distance (record time) over 1500 – 5000-m with the records: 4min 06s at 1500- m, 6min 08s at 2000-m, 9min 23s at 3000-m, and 16 min 30s at 5000-m (Ettema 1966).

$$D_{lim} = a + b \times t_{lim}$$

where "a" is the distance (in meters) that can be run on oxygen reserves and the energy provided by anaerobic metabolism. And "b" is the critical speed, which is the maximum speed compatible with the reconstitution of these reserves by aerobic metabolisms. In Figure 30, "a" is the intercept of the line D lim with the ordinate axis and is equal to 306 meters; b is the slope of the straight-line D-lim and equal to 4.7 m/s. Thus, the time limit at a given speed depends on the difference between this velocity and the maximum velocity maintained with the reconstitution of energy by the oxidative phosphorylation, called by Ettema: "critical speed." Taking the time limits of 4 to 30 minutes, as recommended by Scherrer (1989), who initiated this concept of critical power, it is possible to determine CS from athletes' records. This critical velocity is approximately 10 percent greater than the maximum steady-state lactate velocity (vMLSS).

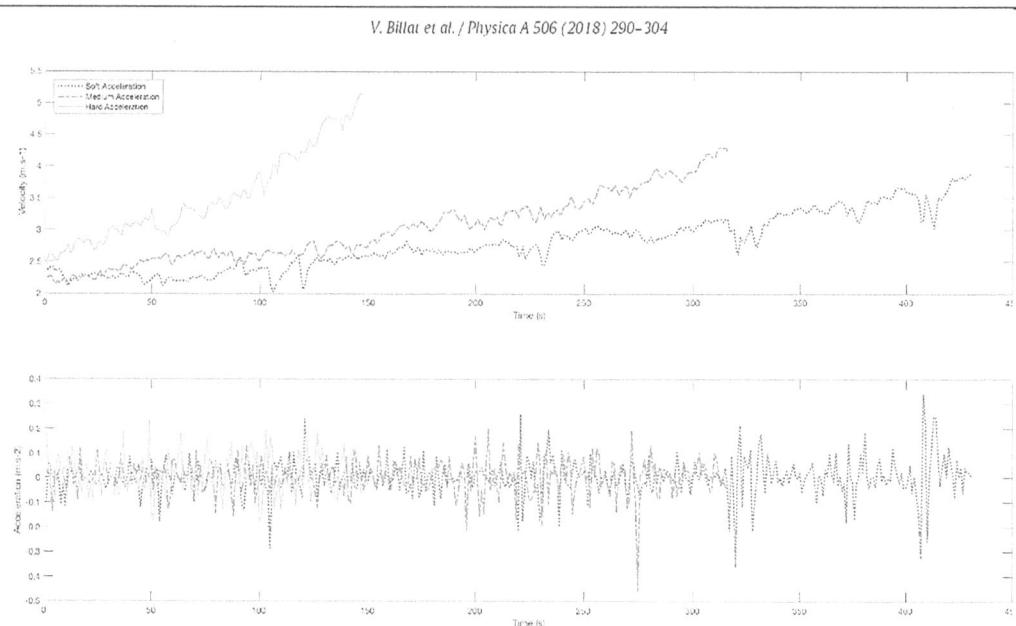

Figure 31. Determination of the CS by the slope of the record distance-time relationship. This runner has a CS of 4.7 m/s, i.e., 17 km/hr or 10.56 mph.

CS is important because it is a physiological value that advanced coaches and physiologists can use to write exercise prescriptions for their athletes. Think of CS as an estimate of where your blood lactate exists while running at a pace that feels stable or at steady-state; we call this the velocity at maximum lactate at steady state (vMLSS). The critical speed is an index which allows, without physiological measurements, an estimate of both the endurance and the anaerobic capacity of a runner. Although, vMLSS is the gold standard for measuring aerobic capacity and is important for the prescription of training for endurance athletes, measuring the vMLSS is not practical because of its time-consuming nature (several days to complete the series of prolonged exercises) and the numerous blood samples. Thus, CS is an interesting and alternative low cost and non-invasive method to prescribe training plans. At www.Billa-Training.com, we use CS for our athletes and incorporate it into their training plans.

Critical speed also helps us to understand that if we run at speeds above the CS (about 90 percent of MAS), we cannot consume the amount of oxygen necessary to resynthesize ATP at the rate needed for muscle contraction. However, between 90 – 100 percent of MAS (between the CS and MAS) VO2 increases again, exponentially. Recall Jerzy Zoladz, a well-known Polish physiologist, has demonstrated that the relationship between VO2 and speed is not linear. He describes inflation of oxygen consumption or a "VO2 excess." Interestingly, this second VO2 phenomenon is not related to the additional mobilization of type IIa muscle fibers. Type IIa fibers are mixed aerobic and anaerobic from their enzymatic machinery. This increase is interpreted as muscular fatigue (inability to maintain constant power). This muscle fatigue is the result of the increase in AMP, IMP, H + ions, and the reduction in creatine phosphate with increased creatine and inorganic phosphates. All these phenomena are described as those of muscular fatigue (Korzeniewski and Zoladz 2006).

MEASUREMENT OF CRITICAL SPEED

Determining your CS is relatively easy and does not require complicated equipment and is best done at a 400-m track. With an adequate warm-up, the idea is to run all out for 3 minutes. Your CS is the speed over the last 30 seconds. More precisely, the average of your speeds over the last 30 seconds is the CS. The distance covered in those 30 seconds is known as your D prime (D'). D' is the extra distance you can cover regardless of your speed above CS. Most runners will attain their CS in 2 minutes of all-out running. The test is as hard as it sounds but think of it as a 180-second investment into your training regimen. Repeat the CS test 2 or 3 times when you are well rested for an accurate result. Remember, this is a measurement of your speed as it **decreases** from your top VO2 max speed, thus it is a speed well below your sprint speed. In theory, you should be able to sustain an effort at CS for about 40 to 60 minutes.

An example of CS in an elite runner is Eliud Kipchoge. In 2017, it was reported that he had a CS of 6.04 m/s and D' of 250 meters. This means that he could run faster than 6.04 m/s, but it doesn't matter if he runs at 6.2 or 6.6 m/s, he will stop from fatigue as soon as he covers 250 meters more than if he ran at his CS of 6.04 m/s for that period. The distance you can cover above CS is fixed no matter how fast or slow you run; this is a fascinating concept that is useful in running.

The question is often asked if you can raise your CS. The short answer is yes. But the more important question to ask is, why do we fatigue at speeds below CS? There are many factors, and they are complex - thermoregulation, the blood supply to the skin, glycogen depletion, lactate threshold, glucose metabolism, injuries, and much more. The moment the muscle cell recognizes low glucose in the blood, a central (brain) feed-forward mechanism will limit the level of exercise. Increasing mitochondrial density is another thing that will improve your performance and CS. Long runs or cycling (sometimes in a fasted state) increases mitochondrial density. Likewise, performing high-intensity intervals such as 30-30s also increase mitochondrial density.

> ## Learning from History
>
> It is interesting to look at historical physiological landmarks that have evolved alongside training methods during the 20th century. These are the ideas that led to concepts like CS and MAS. Today these poorly understood and widespread notions on the internet are an obstacle to those runners questioning traditional the monotony of training methods and lead to overtraining. Here are the historical, scientific concepts in the field of physiology and important steps in the evolution of records and training techniques in cross-country running: the development of MAS, t-lim, and the CS concept.

- 1910 The oxygen consumption (VO2) at exercise begins to be correctly measured.
- 1912 Finnish and Olympic champion Hannes Kolehmainen introduced the split training of breaking the competition distance into 5 to 10 repetitions at the speed of competition: for example, for the 10-km he was running 10 × 1000-m at his competitive pace on 10-km (3 min 05 for 1000-m) or 19 km/hr.
- 1927 Hill A.V develops the concept of maximum oxygen consumption (VO2 max).
- 1920 Pavoo Nurmi (Finland) ran a 14min 36s 5000-m and introduced interval training over short distances (200 – 400-m) inside a slow and long race: 6 × 400m in 60 seconds in a race of 10 to 20 km.
- 1964 The anaerobic ventilatory threshold by Wasserman and McIlroy.
- 1960 Astrand (Swedish physiologist) develops the long interval method: 3 minutes of running at 90 percent of VO2 max and 3 minutes of trotting at 30 – 40 percent of VO2 max.
- 1960 Lydiart (New Zealand), develops the method of short intervals: 15-15s for 30 minutes. Dr. Billat reworked this method in the 2000s by demonstrating that the speeds of 100 and 70 percent of MAS (work and recovery) allowed VO2 max solicitation without lactate accumulation. Similarly, the famous 30-30s at 100 and 50 percent of MAS performed in 1 series (20 repetitions) allowed one to maintain VO2 max throughout the session except for the first 4 repetitions necessary for the rise of VO2 to VO2 max.
- 1966 CS concept by Ettema. This is the speed corresponding to the asymptote of the speed-time relation. Initially, this critical speed was calculated from running at a constant speed between 80 and 110 percent of MAS. It corresponds to speed between the vMLSS speed or the ventilation threshold and MAS. This CS corresponds to the tempo training speed close to the one-hour record speed on fractions of 20 to 40 minutes. This concept was also used to calculate the number of possible repetitions at a given speed by

knowing the CS and anaerobic capacity ADC or Anaerobic Distance Capacity (intercept of the relation distance time or surface of the relation speed-time).

- 1979 Keul and Kinderman established the aerobic (lactate 2mM) and anaerobic thresholds (lactate 4mM).

- 1950 The short intervals of Zatopek and Van Aacken (30 to 50 repetitions of 1 to 1 minute 30 with jogging recovery of the same duration) were run at the anaerobic threshold. Even in the 1950s, Zatopek was using classic interval training. The effectiveness of interval training ran at threshold over short distances and repeated many times is still debated. Example: 100 × 400m in 1 minute and 30 seconds (15 km/hr) with a 200-m jog between each repetition. He ran up to 50-km a day. At that time, it was thought that training needed to be more intensive. Gerschler advocated interval-training at speeds higher than MAS and implemented by 5000-m runners. Siegfried Hermann who practiced this type of training by repeating 30 × 200 meters. Tired of these monotonous rehearsals, he switched to training methods prescribed by Van Aacken, another German doctor and ex-runner who advocated fundamental endurance training (at heart rates lower than 150 bpm). Using this method, Siegfried Hermann made considerable strides in his 5000-m time by running 13min30s in 1966 versus 14min10s in 1960.

- 1980 Jack Daniels develops the concept of MAS. He performed these experiments on treadmills as well as in the field. He developed MAS because of the lack of standard protocols and inconsistencies in testing VO2 max in American runners tested in different laboratories. At that time, VO2 max machines only existed in medical laboratories. For practical and economic reasons, they developed methods to measure MAS in the field. The Canadian Luc Léger (1989) popularized measuring MAS in the field by publishing the University of Montreal Track Test (UMTT). Schools and clubs were flooded with cassettes sold by the physiologists.

The training at this time was based on the MAS:

- Short intervals: 200, 300, or even 400-m or 30-30s to 100-105 percent of MAS alternated by 30-second recoveries between 50 – 70 percent of MAS.
- Long intervals: 1600 – 2000-m at 90 percent of MAS with the total distance equal to double the running distance.

- 1994 Billat demonstrates that the T-lim for MAS has a variability of 25 percent in a population of runners with the same MAS.

- 1985-1995 Lipox Speed and Crossover Point Concept (Brooks and Mercier 1994). The concept of crossover describes the effects of exercise and endurance training on the balance of carbohydrate (CHO) and lipid metabolism during sustained exercise. The crossover point is when the energy output is derived from CHO-derived fuels and predominates over energy derived from fatty acids. Contemporary literature contains data indicating that after endurance training, exercise at low intensities (< or = 45 percent VO2 max) is accomplished with lipids as the primary substrate. This led to the concept of lipox-max. The lipox-max concept is used in training and weight loss in obese subjects. However, the lipox-max concept came into question because of its overdependence on the conditions at the time of measurement and especially the diet.

- 1999 Billat shows that MAS training must consider the time limit at MAS. Indeed, regardless of the time limit at MAS, runners completed five repetitions at MAS with a duration equal to 50 percent of MAS's time limit. This type of training performed once a week (combined with a threshold training) significantly improves MAS in 4 weeks (+ 1.2 km/hr for runners whose MAS was already 19 km/hr).

- 1999 Billat studies the critical velocity at VO2 max. Critical velocity is the highest speed beyond VO2 max. This speed is cl.ose to MAS because it is determined from a succession of independent runs at constant speed running until exhaustion between 90 – 140 percent of MAS.

This critical velocity at VO2 max 15-15s is performed by running short 15-15 type intervals at 90 – 80 percent MAS (for a critical speed at 85 percent of MAS). This type of very short interval-training training allows a runner to tolerate VO2 max for 15 minutes and ensures the progress of master runners (> 45 years old) by improving the maximum steady-state speed of lactate by more than 10 percent and their T-lim over 50 percent.

- 2012 Petot demonstrates that the decrease in speed during a MAS test makes it possible to go beyond the ceiling of VO2 max. This study revived VO2 by making it made it possible to rethink the possibility of increasing the energy at VO2 max, which could be a factor to improve performance.

- 2015 Billat develops the Rabit® test (Running Advisor Billat Training) developed by the BillaTraining.com company in 2015, making it possible to determine the four factors of the performance (Power, Cardiac efficiency, Tolerance to acidosis and Perception) on race distances from 3000-m to the marathon. Performing two workouts a week of 30 minutes (active work) and connecting these themes allow progress at any age and any level of performance.

- 2018 Billat observes that the time limit at VO2 max is not a discriminating factor of performance. This observation is probably also valid for VO2 max, which is only a laboratory artifact. It is necessary to move more towards the maximum power and the force (specific to an activity), which makes it possible to maximally solicit the metabolism synchronously by varying the speed with a sufficient reserve of power. Speed variation is the short-controlled accelerations which are dependent on the strength of the runner. It is the speed reserve that must be improved to be able to run without fatigue or injury. The human runner has the ability to control accelerations (weak to strong) until exhaustion instinctively.

How to estimate the maximal oxygen consumption of an athlete from a race performance from 2000 – 10000-m:

At 5000-m, a time of 14 minutes and 36 seconds gives a speed of 19.32 km/h. By knowing that a 5000-m run at approximately 94 percent of the speed associated with VO2 max (MAS), we will then obtain a speed associated with a VO2 max of MAS = 100/94 × 19, 32 km / h = 20.64 km/h. If we apply the following equation (Léger and Mercier 1984), which makes it possible to calculate VO2 max from a standard energy cost of 3.5 ml/min/kg per speed and distance traveled (km/hr) (between 10 and 20 km/hr). From this, we get the following equation:

$$\text{VO2 max} = 3.5 \times \text{MAS where v is the speed in km/h,}$$
$$\text{VO2 is in ml/min/kg.}$$

We then obtain a VO2 max:

$$\text{VO2 max} = 3.5 \times \text{MAS} = 3.5 \times 20.64 = 72.2 \text{ ml/min/kg}$$

The same calculation is possible from the distances of 2000, 3000, and 10,000 m knowing that with an average endurance (endurance is defined as the ability to use the highest fraction of VO2 max over a given distance or time):

- The 3000-m runs at 96-98 percent MAS
- The 5000-m runs at 94-95 percent MAS
- The 10,000-m runs at 90-92 percent MAS

Keep in mind that many extrapolations miss the mark since VO2 max predicted from MAS is strictly defined only through the detection of a plateau of VO2 max. If there is no plateau determination, this is only a peak speed after the completion of a stress test with steps of 2 – 3 minutes incremented by 1 km/hr.

The classical methods found nowadays on the internet follow this logic of reasoning: *first, you must determine your maximum aerobic speed. Secondly, depending on your goals, choose a race distance. Finally, you must look at the percent of MAS you expect to maintain during this race. The goal is to ensure that the anaerobic system intervenes as little as possible to produce the energy needed for muscle contraction (the energy chains). For each training program, it is necessary to determine the distance of the performance and stick to it.*

This advice is harmful and does not achieve the intended effects. This discourse of monotonous running does not encourage us to attempt variations of speed. We risk burn out from the first kilometers of the marathon. In a philosophical sense, we need to free the sorrowful minds who are afraid to discover these new opportunities for improving performance and especially making these new sensations more enjoyable.

CHAPTER 11 SUMMARY

CONCEPT: Critical speed (CS) is defined as the race pace for any endurance event lasting between 30 and 60 minutes. It also applies to marathon running and other distances. Critical speed is different from MAS. Recall that MAS is the slowest speed from which VO2 is plateaued at a maximum (VO2 max). But applying MAS to a long endurance race such as a marathon, is not applicable in the real-world. This is why the CS concept was developed and is helpful in a marathon if you want to race to your full potential. CS is an essential tool in predicting performance in a marathon, and the runner with the fastest critical speed should theoretically win the race. This speed beyond which it is no longer possible to remain at a stable VO2 without drifting to VO2 max is called the critical speed. The critical speed is an index which allows, without physiological measurements, an estimate of both the endurance and the anaerobic capacity of a subject. The question is often asked if you can raise your CS. The short answer is yes. But what is more important to ask is, why do we fatigue at speeds below CS? There are many factors, and they are complex: thermoregulation, the blood supply to the skin, glycogen depletion, lactate threshold, glucose metabolism, injuries, and much more.

APPLICATION: Determining your CS is much easier than determining your anaerobic or lactate threshold, and no expensive VO2 max or blood lactate analyzers are necessary. A rough estimation of CS is to run 10 – 15 percent below MAS for more than 3 – 5 minutes to reach the reference VO2 max obtained at MAS in a treadmill test. The human runner has the ability to instinctively control accelerations (weak to strong) until exhaustion.

CHAPTER 12

THE REAL MEANING AND PURPOSE OF THRESHOLD TRAINING

THE CHALLENGE IN RUNNING A good marathon is to "tame" the pace, not too slow, but not too fast. Threshold running is one of the most fundamental and productive types of training that runners can do, but many have trouble putting them into practice. Training at threshold means to run at a pace that will accomplish several things: pushing the limits of lactate buildup, energy preservation, prevent overtraining and instilling the confidence that you can hold this pace for long periods. It is best to think about a threshold pace as "comfortably hard" but not too hard. Threshold training has a rather bad reputation because it can be a relatively intense experience.

BENEFITS OF THRESHOLD TRAINING

The benefits of threshold training are both physiological and psychological. The ability to endure the higher intensity of efforts for more extended periods is the goal. Simply, a threshold run is nothing more than a steady twenty-minute run. For example, if your threshold pace is 6 minutes per mile (3:44 min/km), and you run 5-km, this gives you an eighteen-minute threshold effort. At BillaTraining.com, we have a different take on threshold efforts. Threshold efforts should be made on a relatively flat surface in good weather, as the goal is to maintain a steady effort for a long time. Many runners have trouble resisting the urge to turn a threshold run into a time trial. Many runners feel the euphoria during a threshold run and decide to increase the pace because they feel better; it is natural to want to compete against yourself. Elite runners can achieve a threshold pace without outside assistance such as watches or heart rate monitors.

THRESHOLD TRAINING AND MAXIMAL LACTATE AT STEADY STATE (MLSS)

Establishing the proper threshold pace is technically defined as the pace that produces an elevated yet steady state of blood lactate accumulation. MLSS is defined as the highest blood lactate concentration during exercise that can be maintained without a continual blood lactate accumulation. Simply said, the level of lactate in your blood is remaining the same and not increasing. There is a close relationship between the amount of work put into a marathon and the MLSS. Thus, the threshold pace is a little faster than a pace you could maintain for two or more hours, but much slower than a pace you could maintain for thirty minutes. For most runners, your 10-km pace is probably not far off your threshold pace; however, this may be different for an elite runner. It is crucial to keep in mind that the purpose of threshold sessions is to stress the lactate clearance and recycling capabilities of the body. It should not feel hard, but it requires a bit of focus to maintain.

Generally, the anaerobic threshold is 85 – 90 percent of the MAS, which is approximately 80 – 90 percent of your maximum heart rate. The goal of this training is to push the limits of exhaustion and fatigue and adapt the body to sustain a significant effort for as long as possible, despite the lactate surge above 4 mmol/L. Pushing past the threshold will result in muscles that can no longer recycle lactate. A phenomenon called "acidosis" appears and usually occurs after three-quarters of an hour at the threshold. This is the signal for the mandatory drop in performance. Again, the acidosis has nothing to do with lactic acid, rather intracellular acidosis.

THE INTERNET AND THRESHOLD TRAINING PROGRAMS

Threshold training has been around for a long time, but runners and coaches define them differently. Nowadays, everyone consults the internet for training plans, and this is good because it helps more people receive proper coaching.

However, the runner must be aware of the misinformation (fake news) spread over the internet. It tends to look legitimate to an inexperienced runner. A quick internet search shows many different opinions concerning the feeling of different runners on sessions at the anaerobic threshold. Here are some examples of a threshold session that can be found on the internet:

> *Example 1. It's a pace where the concentration of lactic acid in the blood is close to 4 mmol/L, whether you are a beginner or a professional. There are two thresholds aerobic and anaerobic: aerobic threshold = a light pace where the runner is 70 percent of his HRmax (Heart Rate Max) or almost 70 percent of his MAS. We can maintain this pace for several hours. Anaerobic threshold = a stinging pace where the runner is at almost 90 percent of his HR max, between 85 and 90 percent of his MAS. This effort can be maintained from 5 minutes (for the beginner) to almost 1 hour for the high-level runners.*

This is the type of misinformation causing many people to run too fast, eventually leading to overtraining and injuries. If you read further into these claims made by many websites, running seems to require little practice. This is the type of information that confuses what it means to fractionate a session and when a threshold session ends. More confusing, certain workouts are designed to develop speed, while others make it possible to improve fatigue resistance. At a given pace or intensity, we all tend to run too fast, so the risk is that we will have to abbreviate or, even worse, interrupt the session before the finish.

Another favorite explanation about energy usage and running can be found here:

> *Example 2. "Running is an essentially energetic activity. Energy during running can be transported via three ways: namely the aerobic (which uses oxygen), the anaerobic (without oxygen with lactic acid production) and the alactate anaerobic (without oxygen or the production of lactate). The aerobic path corresponds to the lowest effort intensities up to 65 – 75 percent HR max, i.e., endurance. Oxygen is then used by the body to turn glucose into the energy needed to run. The more you increase your running speed, the more your breathing will increase to bring more oxygen and, thus, more energy. Even before our maximum oxygen consumption is reached (the famous VO2 max), a second process has already started.*

There is a transition zone that serves as a bridge between the two channels, commonly called the threshold."

This all sounds legitimate, except that it is wrong on many levels. Several thresholds exist, the aerobic threshold and the anaerobic threshold and everything in between. We use many energy systems while running. We have outlined some of these systems in earlier chapters (and there are more!). Up to the aerobic threshold (65 – 75 percent HR max), you will run with ease without shortness of breath. From this threshold, your breathing increases, and your body gradually accumulate lactate (not lactic acid). Increasing lactate is a good thing as its role is to carry more energy. The lactate concentration remains low and stable around 2 mmol per liter of blood. Beyond the aerobic threshold, we enter the aerobic - anaerobic transition zone. With increasing speed, breathing continues to increase with increasing shortness of breath and an ever-increasing concentration of lactate in the blood up to 4 mmol/l which corresponds to the second threshold, the anaerobic threshold (85 – 88 percent HR max) can usually be held between 30 – 60 minutes. This is where you are at the breaking point. The balance can be broken at any time between the production and reutilization of lactate in the body. Beyond this threshold, the legs burn and become heavier, and you are short of breath, you are in the red.

EVALUATING THE VENTILATORY AND LACTATE "ANAEROBIC" THRESHOLDS

The lactate threshold originated from East German block sports physiology research in the 1960s. This concept was developed in parallel with the ventilatory threshold coined by Stanford cardiologist Karl Wasserman. Ventilation thresholds were first used to diagnose cardiorespiratory pathology in the 1970s and later used in sports. Ventilatory thresholds were considered to be close to the lactate thresholds without the inconvenience of blood sampling, which was complicated in those days because it required a medical doctor. Likewise, measuring gas exchange was expensive and had to be done in a lab. Today, both lactate and ventilatory thresholds can be easily done by anyone and in the field.

Conventionally, the aerobic energy potential is proportional to the fraction of the oxygen consumption at which the runner begins to accumulate lactate.

This accumulation is a corollary to the glycolytic flux that exceeds the possibilities of oxidative phosphorylation, forcing the athlete to support the acids (H + ions) produced by glycolysis. This all occurs inside the muscle cell where enzymes (lactate dehydrogenase) catalyze the conversion of pyruvate into lactate by buffering the H + ions. Methods for evaluating speed thresholds and the percentage of maximum oxygen consumption are based on blood lactate measurement. Anaerobic glycolysis plays a predominant role in the amount of energy compared to aerobic metabolism; H + ion combines with oxygen to form water and carbon dioxide. This is why we speak of the lactate threshold or the gas exchange method for the ventilatory threshold. Multitudes of anaerobic thresholds and test protocols exist (ventilatory or lactate) using the blood lactate concentration. Beyond MAS and VO2 max, which represents the maximum aerobic power that can be sustained at a so-called time-limit (4 – 10 minutes), the lactate threshold speeds are intended to give athlete endurance dimensions. Again, this is the ability to run at speeds as close as possible to MAS without accumulating lactate or hyperventilation.

For fifty years, we considered the maximum oxygen consumption (VO2 max) the testimony of the ability of a runner to transport and use large quantities of oxygen by promoting oxidative phosphorylation and supply ATP. We now know that VO2 max does not predict the winner of a competition based on the same level of performance. This means that the ability to use a large percentage of VO2 max without accumulating lactate is fundamental in sustaining power over long distances. In the same way, the running economy also determines the final performance. David Costill, an American physiologist, demonstrated that a runner with only a VO2 max of 69.7 ml/kg/min could complete a marathon in 2 hours and 8 minutes at 86 percent of his VO2 max. In 1967, this runner could compete with the best in the world. Many physiologists had their athletes starting marathons with the speed corresponding to a lactate concentration between the two thresholds of 2 – 4 mmol/L. But the speed in a marathon is slightly lower than the maximum speed of lactate accumulation. Glycogen depletion and hyperthermia also require the runner to slow down.

The VO2 max of Dr. Costill's runner was likely underestimated because it was measured on a treadmill using an incremented protocol that does not truly reach VO2 max. Several issues exist with using a treadmill. There is a lack of natural propulsion and a rapid increase in speed. When these things happen, this does not give the body time to slow down and adapt and synchronize to our "hybrid engines." Secondly, remember that the difference in marathon performances between 2 hours 6 minutes and 36 seconds and 2 hours and 11 minutes was correlated with the speed over only 1000-m. Therefore, we can speculate that the speed requiring anaerobic glycolysis can also solicit VO2 max. We observed that VO2 max could be determined in the field by a maximal exercise of fewer than three minutes or even during a sprint (Billat, personal data from national and international sprinters taken from the 100-m track in Aix Les Bains, France). We hope you will be able to reflect on your running sensations and their physiological meanings and reconnect with yourself. By doing this, you can manage your race without worrying about pace and listening to your body.

THE PHASES OF AEROBIC AND ANAEROBIC THRESHOLDS

Let's go deeper into what "threshold" truly means in terms of physiological responses. These phases involve complex physiology and understanding aerobic and anaerobic metabolism in the human body is essential to building a successful training regimen. Many trainers and physiologists often talk about aerobic and anaerobic respiration and metabolism as if they are two separate phenomena. Nothing could be further from the truth. Aerobic metabolism can exist in the face of anaerobic metabolism, and vice versa. It is essential to understand the multitude of techniques used to identify anaerobic thresholds (AT). We are often asked why there are so many methods out there for measuring AT. First, one must understand the complex physiology involved, and the other is that there are too many *chefs* in the kitchen! Anaerobic thresholds differ from one person to the next and vary depending on your sport. Methods for measuring AT are premised on the observation and detection of a breakpoint of metabolic parameters such as lactate and ammonia. Most data are taken from ventilation and blood samples in the laboratory and on the field. Remember that AT is useful in the laboratory and training, but less so in the race.

Always keep in mind that the parameters of AT are, in fact, triangular in nature, meaning the evolution of all these parameters can be broken down into three characteristic intensities during a race. This will help us further understand the multitude of proposed techniques to identify anaerobic thresholds and other values, identifying the maximum intensity from which aerobic energy production is completed and then gradually replacing anaerobic mechanisms. The three remarkable phases of the transition of aerobic to primarily anaerobic metabolism can be characterized by an increasing running intensity (speed and slope).

PHASE 1
$VO_2 \leq 40$ PERCENT OF VO_2 MAX

This is a jogging pace, which gradually increases the pace (up to about 150 bpm). At this time, a larger amount of oxygen is extracted, resulting in a smaller fraction in exhaled oxygen (FEO_2). On the other hand, more CO_2 is produced and exhaled, since oxygen is the final acceptor of the H + ion at the end of the respiratory chain in the mitochondria. This is when the fraction of expired CO_2 ($FECO_2$) increases. We observed a linear increase in oxygen consumption (VO_2), ventilation (VE), expired CO_2 volume ($VCO_2 = VE \times FECO_2$), and heart rate. Little or no lactate is formed during this phase. The lactate is immediately oxidized in the muscle fibers' slow type and the heart muscle cells (myocardium). The blood accumulation of lactate is low because the rate of appearance or "Ra" is low (Brooks 1985). Remember that all of this takes place in the mitochondria.

Measuring exhaled oxygen (VO_2) and carbon dioxide (VCO_2), gives a value called the respiratory quotient (VCO_2/VO_2). The respiratory quotient (R) gives us an estimate of the percentage of energy derived from glycogen (carbohydrates) or lipids (fatty acids). RQ = CO_2 eliminated/O_2 consumed. An RQ of 0.7 denotes that most of our energy is coming from lipids, an RQ of 1.0 denotes that our energy is mainly from glycogen. Realize that our bodies are always using both lipids and carbohydrates for energy. From an energy standpoint, when the respiratory quotient (RQ) is low at 0.7 – 0.8, we are primarily using our aerobic metabolism. This important use of free fatty acids (resulting from ß oxidation) also has an inhibitory effect on glycolysis, sparing muscle glycogen. This happens in the Krebs cycle via citrate, which inhibits pyruvate oxidation and the activity of two glycolytic enzymes: glycerol dehydrogenase and phosphofructokinase. Running slowly does not allow you to save glycogen or develop the ability to build a capacity to increase glycolysis to run faster.

At lower running speeds, the slow-twitch muscle fibers are highly recruited. The glycolytic inhibition induced by the metabolism of free fatty acids is a result of the lower production of lactate and an increase in its oxidation to pyruvate. This process is favored by the H-LDH isoenzymes of type I slow-twitch muscle fibers. **No matter your fitness level, the marathon, and all long-distance events should be run at variable speeds around a medium to hard pace to avoid early depletion of glycogen and neuro-muscular fatigue**. Doing so would lead to the double penalty of increasing the energy cost and over-consumption of oxygen per meter run. However, we know that if you increase your stride frequency for the same slow speed, more fast-twitch fibers (type IIa) will be stimulated by accelerated neuromuscular excitation.

Again, in the context of an incremental protocol, as running speed increases, more type I (oxidative) fibers and perhaps some type II (glycolytic) fibers are mobilized. This causes an increase in ATP utilization. The products of ATP metabolism increase adenosine monophosphate (AMP), ADP, ammonium ion (NH4 +) and inorganic phosphate (Pi). The accumulation of these metabolites decreases the inhibitory effect of citrates on phosphofructokinase activity (PFK), promoting a higher rate of glycolysis. Since the oxidation of free fatty acids is still high, some inhibition of pyruvate is still present. Therefore, there is an imbalance between pyruvate production and oxidation, some of which will be reduced to lactate (Brooks 1985). This explains the slight elevation of the blood lactate from 1 to about 3 mmol/L. Thus, it is due to an excess of pyruvate and not hypoxia (deficiency of oxygen) in the mitochondria of the muscle fiber cells that lactate increases while running at 40 percent of VO2.

PHASE 2
VO2 = 40 – 60 PERCENT OF VO2 MAX

With the acceleration of running speeds up to 40 – 60 percent of VO2 max, VO2 and HR always increase linearly. The participation of Type IIa and IIb fast-twitch fibers are increasing as well as increased use of ATP. As stated above, the increased use of ATP reduces the inhibitory effect of citrate on PFK activity and improves the glycolysis rate. Added to this is the activity of the M-LDH isoenzyme of type II fibers, which leads to increased lactate production and increased ventilation (VE) to compensate for metabolic acidosis. The accumulation of lactate during this phase is from about 2 – 4 mmol/L according to the muscular typology of the runner, which is the percentage of slow fibers (80 percent for a highly trained runner) and fast fibers. This slight accumulation causes a reduction in the use of fats and an increase in the use of muscle glycogen. Lactate ($C_3H_6O_3$) being completely dissociated in the human body into lactate and hydrogen ions ($C_3H_5O_3$-H), and it is buffered in the cell by the bicarbonate ion (HCO_3)

$$HCO_3- + H+ \rightarrow H_2O + CO_2$$

This results in excess CO_2 that ventilation "eliminates" by increasing respiratory rate, or VE, and therefore VCO_2. The increase of VE and VCO_2 is higher than that of VO_2, causing a disproportionate increase of the ventilatory equivalent for oxygen: VE/VO_2 and the respiratory quotient, R (VCO_2/VO_2). The system does not consume as much oxygen as is required by oxidative phosphorylation (to replace the ATP used). The increase in VE causes a lower oxygen extraction per volume of ventilated air, and this is why the fraction of expired oxygen (FEO_2) is increasing. The beginning of this second phase is therefore characterized by the increase of FEO_2, without the corresponding decrease of $FECO_2$. This corresponds to the ventilatory anaerobic threshold (Wasserman 1973).

PHASE 3
VO_2 = 65 – 90 PERCENT OF VO_2 MAX

When the running speed increases to 65 and 90 percent of VO_2 max, the linear increase of VO_2 and HR continues until the MAS, where these parameters reach a plateau. It should be noted that some authors (Conconi 1982) report anaerobic threshold by the slight deflection of the heart rate, leaving its linear progression as a function of the stroke speed. This serves as a basis for the Conconi test, which identifies a deflection of the heart rate at the lactate threshold of 4 mmol/L (Figure 32).

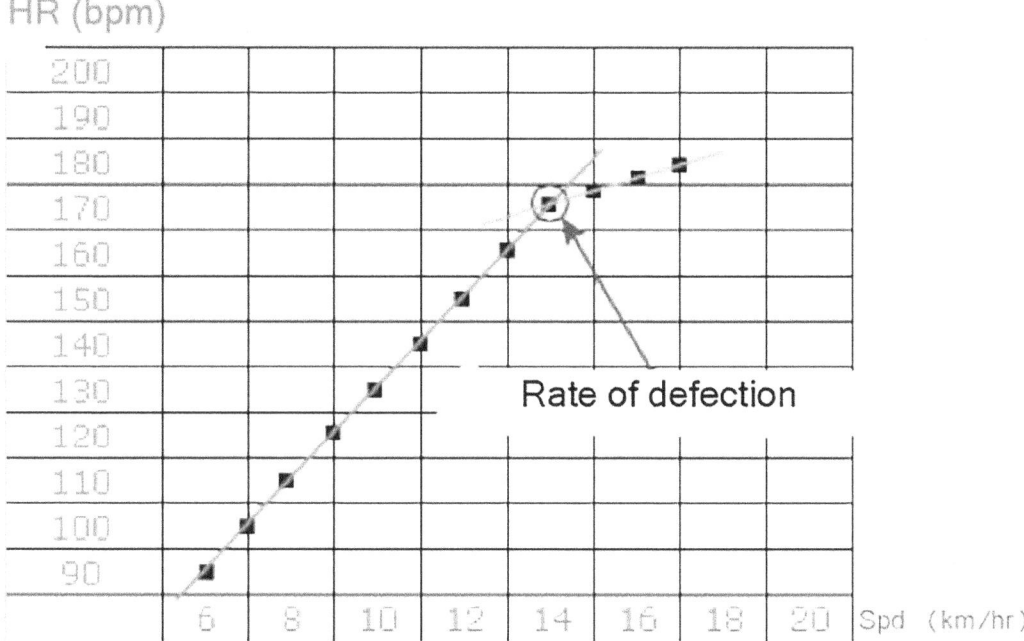

Figure 32. Determination of the deflection point of the Conconi heart rate.

At the beginning of this phase, the blood lactate is about 4 mmol/L. This value increases exponentially until the runner reaches his MAS; we regularly see lactate values higher than 8 mmol/L. Of course, beyond this speed, the accelerated rate of lactate production is due to the solicitation of anaerobic glycolysis, which brings the surplus of energy necessary to accelerate the speed. The latter is said to be "supra-maximal" when it is higher than the maximum aerobic speed and approaches VO2 max. Between 65 and 90 percent of VO2 max, we observe several things: an accumulation of lactate, an accelerated increase of the respiratory rate, and a continuous increase of VCO2 compensating the increased accumulation of blood lactate. Keep in mind this occurs due to a break in the equilibrium between the rate of lactate formation and recycling. At this stage, however, hyperventilation can no longer compensate for the increase in blood lactate. The decrease in FECO2 (exhaled air fraction in CO2) is then observed, while FEO2 continues to increase. This is all complex physiology, but hopefully, you gain an appreciation of the process.

Seldom considered, when we hyperventilate, significant amounts of oxygen are used by the accessory muscles involved in hyperventilation (intercostal, scalenes, etc.) Thus, a portion of VO2 is no longer available to the heart muscle (myocardium) or skeletal muscles demanding more oxygen. The beginning of this third phase is therefore characterized by a sudden increase in blood lactate starting from 4 ± 2 mmol/L by a decrease in FECO2 and marked hyperventilation. More Type II fibers are recruited as the intensity of the race increases. Due to the M-LDH isoenzyme pattern of these fibers, lactate levels continue to rise, thus causing a further decrease in lipolysis (fat burning) activity.

ANAEROBIC THRESHOLDS AND TESTING PROTOCOLS

There are many testing protocols for AT's. The standard for measuring AT involves using an expensive respiratory gas analyzer in a laboratory or the field. The analyzers that we use in the field cost well over 40,000 Euros. Blood lactate and heart rate protocols are not precise and only approximate AT. Measuring blood lactate is invasive and does not guarantee optimal precision since lactate concentrations vary between runners. Heart rate is also a popular method used to measure anaerobic thresholds. Heart rate is not entirely accurate in measuring AT, but it is simple and gives us a ballpark figure. By measuring heart rate data during maximal exercise, we can look for deflections in the heart rate, and this corresponds to the anaerobic threshold. This happens when your hybrid battery gives up, and the recycling of lactate is no longer efficient or possible.

To calculate AT using heart rate: subtract 220 minus your age and multiply the result by 0.935.

For example, for a 40-year-old man: 220 - 40 = 180 × 0.935 = 168 bpm.

THE CONCONI TEST

The Conconi test is often used on websites that explain "how to determine the anaerobic threshold?" Conconi described the AT by the slight deflection of the heart rate, leaving its linear progression as a function of the stroke speed. This serves as a basis for the Conconi test, which identifies a deflection of the heart rate at the lactate threshold of 4 mmol/L (figure 32). To perform the Conconi test, you need a heart rate monitor that can record your HR, which you can then transfer to a graph or computer software. After a warm-up of twenty minutes at 60 percent HR max, increase your running speed by 0.5 km/h every

200-m or 1 km/h every 400-m until the end of the effort. The goal is to correlate your HR with your running speed. According to Professor Conconi, the heart rate increases linearly during an effort up to the point of inflection (also called deflection rate), identifying the transition zone between the aerobic and anaerobic pathways. Then there is a point of sagging heart rate that represents the anaerobic threshold.

Recall that the Franceso Conconi is an Italian sports doctor who was involved in introducing erythropoietin (EPO) to many sports, including running and cycling in the 1980s. His research focused on developing techniques to detect EPO, but most of his training science was a decoy for developing EPO use in sports. In the 1980s and 1990s, he and several of his assistants (Michele Ferrari) were charged with doping activities. Unfortunately, these chains of events set back exercise science for many years, and we are just getting back to untainted science.

In 2005, we studied athletes with large systolic ejection volumes (SEV). In these athletes, the SEV did not reach a plateau, making it possible to increase cardiac output without an increase in heart rate. When this happens, less oxygen is consumed by the myocardium. This is important because an important concept in cardiac physiology is that the heart always feeds itself first. The heart uses the most oxygen (11 percent at rest) and more than double that (25 percent) when the VO2 max is reached. We use MVO2 to designate the VO2 of the myocardium. At rest, the MVO2 is about 11 percent, while at VO2 max, it is around 25 percent. Thus, the demand for oxygen is highly dependent on the work of the heart, namely, the heart rate. We can already see that the difference in the methods used is based on the variable definitions and modes of identification of lactate, cardiac, or ventilatory breakpoints.

FLAWS IN ANAEROBIC THRESHOLDS

Many authors have remarked that training in a zone of 65 – 90 percent of VO2 max at a constant pace training pushes the anaerobic metabolism to a higher VO2 max without lactate accumulation resulting in a supposed increased endurance. These flawed ideas are based on the belief that the "onset" of anaerobic metabolism begins at higher percentages of VO2 max between 65 and 90 percent. Intermittent training improves the ventilatory threshold more than continuous pace training and shows no differences in the lactate threshold. High-intensity interval training studies of 8 weeks have shown that there is a dissociation of the effects of the interval-training on the ventilatory and lactate response.

The central nervous system (CNS) can affect these adaptations to acceleration and sudden deceleration, leading to a possible dissociation in lactate and ventilation thresholds. This CNS theory has been shown in patients with glycogen storage disease, McArdle's syndrome. These patients have a deficiency in muscle phosphorylase, resulting in the inability to degrade their muscle glycogen and often die from extremely low blood sugars in their sleep. During exercise, these patients do not increase in their blood lactate, but hyperventilation appears from a certain intensity of muscle exercise (Hagberg 1982). A cycling study obtained similar results in healthy subjects while cycling in a state of glycogen depletion (Hughes 1982). This means that if we test a runner 1 or 2 days after a session performed at intensities close to 80 – 100 percent VO2 max (preferably using carbohydrates, with a respiratory quotient equal to 1), it is highly likely that the "lactate threshold" will not appear exactly at the same speed. Even more, if we fat adapt these individuals, their lactate thresholds will be different as well.

Nevertheless, all the methods and techniques for the detection of ventilatory or lactate thresholds come from triangular stress protocols, during which the running speed is progressively accelerated every 30 seconds, or 1, 2, 3, or 4 minutes, from a few meters up to 2 km per hour. The choice of duration and speed increments is not without impact on the results (Yoshida 1984).

LACTATE TERMINOLOGIES AND THE AEROBIC-ANAEROBIC THRESHOLDS

Since the original concept of anaerobic threshold by the American cardiologist Karl Wasserman, the debate over the choice of parameters and its methods have been very animated during the last fifteen years.

The basis of these controversies concern:

1. The role of hypoxia on the lactate threshold.

2. Correspondence of lactate and ventilatory thresholds.

To give you a glimpse of pointless scientific articles that have debated the "true anaerobic threshold," we can reference these publications:

- The significance of the aerobic-anaerobic transition for the determination of workload intensities during endurance training (Kinderman 1979).

- The aerobic-anaerobic threshold (Mader and Heck 1986).

- Skinner and McLellan, 1980 "OBLA" (Onset of Blood Lactate Accumulation).

- "OPLA" (Onset of Plasma Lactate Accumulation) or onset of accumulation of plasma lactate (Farrel 1979).

- "Lactate Threshold" (Ivy 1980), "Lactate turning point" (Davis 1983).

- "The individual anaerobic threshold" or IAT (Stegmann 1981).

These are all confusing terminologies that describe the abrupt evolution of lactatemia as a function of exercise. The onset of plasma lactate accumulation (OPLA), maximal lactate steady state, lactate threshold, anaerobic threshold, the onset of blood lactate accumulation, individual anaerobic threshold, lactate threshold-1 (LT1), lactate threshold-2 (LT2), and there are more. All these lactate thresholds were determined by tests using progressive increases in intensity (VAMEVAL tests). The **intermediate** values of a lactate threshold test determine "the aerobic-anaerobic transition zone" (Keul 1978). The choice of the protocol, and the duration of the stages, plays a key role in the values obtained from the anaerobic threshold tests (Yoshida 1984). For example, Stegmann and Kindermann (1982) observed that subjects performing an exercise at the threshold of 4 mmol/L could not support more than a few minutes at steady state. However, these same subjects performed a stepwise 30-minute test in a state of lactate equilibrium when the exercise corresponds to their threshold previously determined by the method described above. Thus, the duration of the effort and intensity cannot be separated. Indeed, the maximum stable state defining an intensity for which the lactatemia is stabilized as a function of time after the appearance of the early lactate characterizes the maximal intensity of exercise for which the appearance of lactate in the blood is equivalent to its disappearance (Brooks 1986).

Then we started thinking outside of the box: why use these notions of artificially determined physiological thresholds during artifact protocols that have nothing to do with the real race? All these thresholds were therefore determined during a progressively accelerated treadmill test, which has little do with how you are going to run in a race. A study of high-level marathoners over a distance of 10 km found that lactate levels at the end of a 10-km race in elite marathoners were 10 ± 3 mmol/L in the males 8.7 ± 4.1 for the females (Billat 2001).

LIES, MYTHS, AND THE INTERNET

Runners are often flooded by imprecisions found on internet blogs. For example, it is often taken as gospel that when the lactate concentration reaches 4mmol/L, it is defined as the anaerobic threshold and used as a baseline corresponding to their training level. Many blogs state that the only way to precisely measure the anaerobic threshold is through several blood tests. This also could not be farther from the truth.

The physiological zone of the anaerobic threshold can be ascertained by performing moderate-rate fractional sessions where the effort's intensity is controlled based on the maximum heart rate. This usually occurs at approximately 90 – 92 percent of the maximum heart rate. Surprisingly enough, the heart rate turns out to be the miracle indicator of the anaerobic threshold. The threshold corresponds to the race pace that can be held for 50 – 60 minutes. We give the runner a better notion of threshold by telling the runner that he/she can free themselves by staying in a zone close to the maximum heart rate, or what we would call a "medium plus" sensation zone.

Runners looking for precision on the internet will be disappointed. Take this blog, for example: *"You can succeed in tempo without precisely knowing your anaerobic threshold. Just make sure to be below rather than above by taking a margin with a pace a little slower than a 10-km pace that you can hold for about 1 hour, that is to say, a pace where you are on a good pace but still comfortable, without having shortness of breath and high heart rate ... All these elements are signs that show you what the pace is at the anaerobic threshold! I hope this helps you!"*

Yes, help yourself, and the web will help you!

But if we persevere on the internet, we discover that the "new method" of using lactate is in fashion rather than the threshold. *"The blog author announces a new goal of "Lactate Shuttle" sessions in order "to teach" the body to use lactate as a fuel and to spare glycogen and incidentally to reduce acidosis. It is a marathon preparation-oriented session for its goal on the ability to save glycogen. It is a physiological process to circulate lactate in the body, especially between muscle fibers."*

It should be remembered that anaerobic metabolism is a physiological process called glycolysis, which takes place inside muscle cells producing ATP, pyruvate, and H + ions, the proton responsible for the acidosis of muscles and blood. However, too often acidosis, lactate concentration, and blood pH are confused. First, we have already mentioned that lactic acid cannot exist in the human body. Acidosis or increased blood pH is an increased concentration of H + ions (acidic protons). It is considered that blood lactate higher than 4 mmol/L is responsible for impeding increasing exercise intensities and that it is also responsible for "pain" experienced at higher intensities. At most, this pain is a "tingling" sensation in the cheeks and legs, provided you run 400-m all out, inducing a blood lactate level greater than 12 mmol/L. However, this concept of lactate clearance as it relates to a real race is premised on finding a balance in the variations of pace. Lactate can, therefore, leave the muscle cell carried by proteins called monocarboxylate transporter (MCT), which increases with training and is used for energy metabolism. These proteins are significantly improved by training. Endurance training increases the expression of MCT1 with varying effects on MCT4.

MCT transporters function to bring lactate to cells in the liver where lactate is converted into glucose and in the heart where it is used directly as fuel. Likewise, lactate can migrate from fast-twitch muscle fibers where it is produced to slow-twitch muscle fibers where it is recycled to pyruvic acid. Pyruvic acid moves to the mitochondria and enters the Krebs cycle and then the respiratory chain for the regeneration of a large amount of ATP per molecule of glucose (38 ATP). This shuttle provides fuel to the muscle fibers and heart (pyruvate from the lactate transported), which spares glycogen. The H + ions feed the respiratory chain that uses the H+ with the oxygen to produce ATP, all the while decreasing acidosis. However, here again, the pace recommended improving this shuttle process is based on … the lactate threshold! Certainly, the most effective pace to utilize lactate is the aerobic threshold called LT1 (about 78 percent of the MAS). The argument is that up to this speed, lactate remains practically at the resting value and that beyond this speed, the lactate level increases with a subsequent phase of stabilization in duration as long as the pace does not increase or does not exceed the anaerobic threshold or LT2 (about 88 percent of the MAS). Finally, it amounts to relying again on the famous aerobic and anaerobic threshold by introducing the notion of duration and steady-state running in an interesting way without getting away from the goal.

More interestingly, an increase in blood lactate will activate lactate clearance via a decrease of running speed in 2 phases for this session:

1. In the first phase, the rate of lactate production is increased. The first phase's pace and duration should be at those values where we reach a lactate concentration of 4 mmol/L. Note that this pace is the LT2, the last speed, or the lactate level that can still be controlled. Here again, is the question of relying on an anaerobic threshold determination with reference to a triangular treadmill test.

2. The second phase is about maximal lactate utilization. This phase must be run at LT1, the most favorable pace to reduce the lactate production rate to a minimum.

Thus, the level of metabolic clearance of lactate is an important factor in the elimination of lactate and provides a means of describing the interactions between the level of elimination, blood lactate concentration, and blood flow. The removal of lactate would be increased by:

- Acceleration of the elimination of blood lactate by other organs (heart and liver) (Hermansen and Vaage 1977).

- Increased elimination by inactive skeletal muscles (Hermansen and Stenvold 1972).

- Increase in the elimination of lactate produced by glycolytic fibers by oxidative fibers (Connett 1986).

- Training reduces lactate production in the first few minutes of maximal exercise under steady-state conditions (Favier 1986).

- Temperature increases at 50 percent VO2 max would decrease the concentration of early lactate (Pendergast 1983).

In summary, the MLSS is defined as the highest lactate level that can be maintained over time without continuous accumulation of lactate in the blood. However, lactate has been reported showing high variability between individuals (2 – 8 mmol/L) in blood capillaries. The fate of increased lactate clearance in trained individuals has been attributed mainly to oxidation in the active muscle and gluconeogenesis in the liver. The transport of lactate into and out of cells is facilitated by proteins called monocarboxylate transporters (MCT). The stabilized lactatemia corresponds to this power or critical speed of between 2.2 and 6.8 mmol/L depending on the athlete. The calculation of power at the maximum steady-state velocity of lactatemia may not truly reflect the lactate's maximum stable state (over time). This is why at BillaTraining.com, we prefer to underestimate the maximum steady-state velocity of lactate (Billat 1994c) rather than overestimate it by evaluating the lactic threshold by traditional triangular protocols.

CHAPTER 12 SUMMARY

CONCEPT: The real meaning for threshold sessions is to learn to "tame" the pace, not too slowly, but not too fast. Threshold running is one of the most fundamental and productive types of training that runners can do, but many runners have trouble putting them into practice. Training at threshold basically means to run at a pace that will accomplish several things: pushing the limits of lactate buildup, energy preservation, prevent overtraining, and instilling the confidence that you can hold this pace for long periods. It is best to think about a threshold pace as "comfortably hard" but not too hard. Threshold training has a rather bad reputation because it can be a relatively intense experience.

APPLICATION: The benefits of threshold training are both physiological and psychological. The ability to endure greater intensity of effort for more extended periods is the goal. Simply, a threshold run is nothing more than a steady twenty-minute run. For example, if your threshold pace is 6 minutes per mile (3:44 min/km), and you run a 5-km distance, this gives you an eighteen-minute threshold effort. At BillaTraining.com, we have a different take on threshold efforts. Threshold efforts should be made on a relatively flat surface in good weather, as the goal is to maintain a steady effort for a long time. Many runners have trouble resisting the urge to turn a threshold run into a time trial. Many runners feel the euphoria during a threshold run and decide to increase the pace because they feel better; it is natural to want to compete against yourself. Expert runners can achieve a threshold pace alone, without any outside assistance such as watches or heart rate monitors.

CHAPTER 13
AGING AND MINIMALISTIC ACCELERATION TRAINING

We all desire to be able to run and train into our later years, but with age, we lose several physiologic mechanisms. For example, our ability to recover our muscles is not the same as when we were in our 20's. At BillaTraining.com, we teach our master's and older runners to train using a qualitative-minimalistic approach. The word "qualitative training" means to use your senses, run by feel, don't try to put numbers on it. The goal is the know your body when running easy, medium, and hard efforts. By practicing qualitative-minimalistic training, you will instinctively train without putting undue stress on the body.

MARATHON PARTICIPATION IS INCREASING

With age changing in our physiology, it is ironic that many people decide to run a marathon after the age of forty. Most are hoping for transformation, an increase in longevity, and wellness. Interestingly, the rise of the modern fitness industry is a twentieth-century phenomenon as the general population before us did not regularly exercise. The growing interest in the benefits of sport and well-being has led researchers (Lepers and Cattagni 2012) to analyze the effects of age and gender on performance during the New York City marathon. They concluded that the master's athlete's performance increased more than younger ones, meaning they saw more improvements in older compared with younger runners. Forty percent of New York marathon participants run regularly, as compared to 25 percent in the Paris marathon. In both the New

York and Paris marathons, more than 50 percent of male athletes were over forty years old. This phenomenon has experienced tremendous growth. Between 1980 and 1989, the participation rate of men over forty in the legendary New York marathon was 36 percent. Since 1989 it has exploded to 53 percent, meaning that one out of two runners were over forty. Women follow nearly the same trend. Today, 4 out of 10 participants, are forty years of age or older.

The performances of the 30-year-old marathoners have remained stable, while those in the master's categories continue to improve. To put this in perspective, for an average marathon of 3 hours and 50 minutes in the 1980s, men aged 65 to 69 saw their time decrease by eight minutes in the 1990s and another seven minutes in the between 2000s! This is a total decrease of fifteen minutes, resulting in an average time of only 3 hours and 35 minutes. We observed the same trend in women over thirty years; the 55-59 age group have, for example, reduced their marathon time by forty-one minutes, with a time of 3 hours and 32 minutes. In addition, the performance gap between men and women in the same age group seems to be stabilizing across all age groups. Current data suggest that age-related physiological decline is similar for both sexes. The research is showing that the average time is improving because of the influx of these new participants. We are seeing new generations of runners who are motivated to improve their health through better nutrition and training smarter.

PHYSIOLOGY AND OLDER RUNNERS

One of the first things humans lose with age is the quick muscle control we had as kids. This is due to the nervous system changes; the myelin sheaths surrounding the axons are gradually degraded. Brain chemistry changes decrease the production of certain neurotransmitters (the chemical molecules that transmit messages from one neuron to another). Brain dopamine is decreased and partially responsible for a decline in mobility and attention. Recent studies (Tintignac 2015) show that this loss of muscle mass with age, called sarcopenia, is partially due to disruption of the high-frequency neuromuscular junctions. This is one reason our sprint is not as robust as in our younger years. This decrease of the nerve firing rate is the leading cause of power loss in our running speeds; an excellent example is that it becomes difficult to have a high cadence (160 – 180) or to be able to sprint over 15 mph (25 kph). By integrating accelerations of 10 seconds, starting from a zone of average speed and repeating them ten times every 3 minutes, for example, helps to avoid musculoskeletal and cardiovascular stress.

Qualitative training based on accelerations and decelerations helps to curb the decrease in strength and muscle mass with aging. To improve performance into your forties and beyond, we must highlight the subtleties of personalized and qualitative training by optimizing your power and, therefore, your VO2 max. Just like the muscular system, the cardiovascular and respiratory systems suffer the effects of aging. VO2 max is an indicator of aerobic performance, but also a strong predictor of longevity and mortality (Hawkins 2003). A study by Shvartz and Reibold in 1990 reviewed 62 articles measuring the VO2 max of healthy adults in the United States, Canada, and seven European countries. It came up with a classification of VO2 max with age (Figure 33).

WOMEN

Age (years)	Very poor	Poor	Fair	Average	Good	Very good	Excellent
20-24	< 27	27-31	32-36	37-41	42-46	47-51	>51
25-29	< 26	26-30	31-35	36-40	41-44	45-49	>49
30-34	< 25	25-29	30-33	34-37	38-42	43-46	>46
35-39	< 24	24-27	28-31	32-35	36-40	41-44	>44
40-44	< 22	22-25	26-29	30-33	34-37	38-41	>41
45-49	< 21	21-23	24-27	28-31	32-35	36-38	>38
50-54	< 19	19-22	23-25	26-29	30-32	33-36	>36
55-59	< 18	18-20	21-23	24-27	28-30	31-33	>33
60-65	< 16	16-18	19-21	22-24	25-27	28-30	>30

MEN

Age (years)	Very poor	Poor	Fair	Average	Good	Very good	Excellent
20-24	< 32	32-37	38-43	44-50	51-56	57-62	>62
25-29	< 31	31-35	36-42	43-48	49-53	54-59	>59
30-34	< 29	29-34	35-40	41-45	46-51	52-56	>56
35-39	< 28	28-32	33-38	39-43	44-48	49-54	>54
40-44	< 26	26-31	32-35	36-41	42-46	47-51	>51
45-49	< 25	25-29	30-34	35-39	40-43	44-48	>48
50-54	< 24	24-27	28-32	33-36	37-41	42-46	>46
55-59	< 22	22-26	27-30	31-34	35-39	40-43	>43
60-65	< 21	21-24	25-28	29-32	33-36	37-40	>40

Figure 33. Classification of VO2 max (ml/kg/min) values with age based on 62 items measuring VO2 max of healthy adults in the United States, Canada, and European countries. While some cross-sectional studies show a linear decline of about 7 – 10 percent in VO2 max every 10 years (Wilson and Tanaka 2000), longitudinal studies show that this decline accelerates with advancing age, mainly in men (Hawkins and Wiswell 2003).

A closer look at VO2 max shows that it depends on three variables: the maximum heart rate (HR max), the stroke volume (SV), and the arteriovenous difference in oxygen (DavO2). A famous physiologist named Adolf Fick came up with an equation that relied on the observation that the uptake of oxygen in the peripheral tissues is equal to the product of the blood flow to the tissues and the arterial-venous difference of oxygen; he was able to derive VO2 max. He showed that oxygen consumption in the human body is highly dependent on the HR, SV, and arterial – venous difference in oxygen (A – V difference). The calculation is quite complicated, but the point is that with age, HR, SV, and A – V difference decrease. Lowering one of these factors without raising another will ultimately lower VO2 max and performance decreases (Ogawa 1992).

THE FICK EQUATION:

$$VO2 = HR \times SV \times (Da\text{-}vO2)$$

or VO2 is the oxygen consumption (in L/min), HR is in beats per minute, SV is the systolic ejection volume from the heart (in mls of blood per heartbeat) and, the A – V difference. Da-vO2 is used in academics to denote the A – V difference. It is better explained by saying it is the difference in oxygen concentration between the arterial blood (in the muscle) and venous blood (which leaves the muscle).

HR max undeniably decreases with aging (Gellish 2007). In theory, HR max predictably decreases according to the popular Astrand equation (220 – age) or the Karvonen equation (210 - 0.65 × age in years). Therefore, being able to increase one's heart rate with age is important. Recall the story of one-hundred and five-year-old Robert Marchand whose HR max is 135, and VO2 max is 40. Acceleration training prevented the fall of his maximum heart rate. For a given exercise intensity, an older runner will have a higher HR for a given effort (relative to intensity) than a younger runner to compensate for the concomitant decrease in SV during exercise (Fleg 1995). With age, a decrease in myocardial contractility and systolic ejection volume is observed due to a diminished number of cardiac myocytes (cardiac muscle cells), myocardial elasticity, and response to sympathetic stimulation (Shih 2011). However, the decrease in HR max during aging remains the primary mechanism of maximal cardiac output impairment during exercise, thus reducing the maximum oxygen uptake (VO2 max). This is the main factor of increased cardiac output (SV × HR), a central factor of VO2 max.

It is essential to highlight that VO2 max decreases with the loss of muscle mass (sarcopenia). Sarcopenia is not preventable as we age; it is more of a question of decreasing the rate at which it occurs. The decrease in lean body mass and the increase in body fat play an important role in decreasing VO2 max. In contrast, the maintenance of lean body mass and muscle strength appears to maintain VO2 max. At the muscle level, oxidative capacity and capillary density decrease with age, reducing muscle oxygen consumption and consequently, the A – V difference during exercise. All of this goes back to the Fick equation discussed above.

ACCELERATION BASED TRAINING

To study the effects of age on the skeletal and cardiac muscle, researchers at the INSERM laboratory (Launay 2017) studied the effect of acceleration training in rats aged equivalent to eighty human years over 8 weeks (two sessions per week). The results showed an improvement in performance but also VO2 max. Also, increases in cardiac hypertrophy, strength, and muscle mass was observed. Activation of a pathway called mTOR was observed. These results provide new insights into the effectiveness of acceleration-based training protocols. The difficulty of conducting such experiments (cost, installation, etc.) now leads us to research centered on the interpretation of your optimal speed variation in different conditions of distance, shape, and environment.

In these older rats, our new acceleration-based training model improves performance, oxidative capacity, heart function, muscle mass, and mechanical skeletal stability with just 20 – 30 minutes of effort, divided into three sessions during the day, two days a week, for two months. The take-home point is that accelerations are an important stimulus of training. They can induce cardiac and molecular training adaptations in skeletal muscle, thus improving both power and endurance.

The improvement of peak VO2 max in aged rats over six weeks using our acceleration protocol is especially significant because it slows and even reverses the decrease in maximal aerobic power associated with age. However, we know that VO2 max is correlated with life expectancy. Using a meta-analysis (Huang 2005) reported that three sessions of moderate-intensity per week (60 – 70 percent VO2 max) for twenty weeks improved VO2 max in humans. The speed and distance traveled in acceleration-based training were increased in just four weeks in our study, again suggesting that acceleration training induces both cardiovascular and muscle adaptations.

Acceleration-based training induces physiological cardiac remodeling characterized by concentric hypertrophy and systolic optimization, a function evaluated by the systolic ejection fraction. An increase in left ventricle thickness also reported after resistance training (Barauna 2008), occurs through repeated blood pressure elevations during exercise sessions. Our results from acceleration-based training in older rats showed preserved function of the soleus and gastrocnemius muscle efficiency, suggesting that acceleration-based training could reduce this loss of fast-twitch muscle fibers. Indeed, muscle strength depends both on the muscular typology and the size of the fiber. The trained soleus' greater strength suggests a higher number of fast fibers or a higher muscle fiber size. This research's importance is the decrease in skeletal muscle efficiency related to the loss of fast-twitch muscle fibers (Lecarpentier 1998), which are involved in the bone strength and induced by muscular sarcopenia (Witard 2016). Further investigation is needed to clarify this point and understand the molecular mechanisms involved.

The causes of sarcopenia during skeletal aging are multifactorial and complex. Inflammation, oxidative stress, hormones, protein intake, protein synthesis, and damage to DNA are all related to muscle loss. To identify the factors by which acceleration-based training can counteract the effects of aging, we have shown that this new acceleration-based training can activate the pathways of muscle hypertrophy (IGF1R/Akt /mTOR). In conclusion, we have proposed a new mode of acceleration-based training that can counterbalance age-related disability (Figure 34) and trigger cellular and molecular mechanisms to improve cardiac and skeletal function. Speed variation is a better stimulus for training biological adaptations rather than constant duration and intensity. Varying speed is an important factor when preparing customized training protocols for older people. In addition, such short training periods could be an easy long-term plan to aging well and staying healthy.

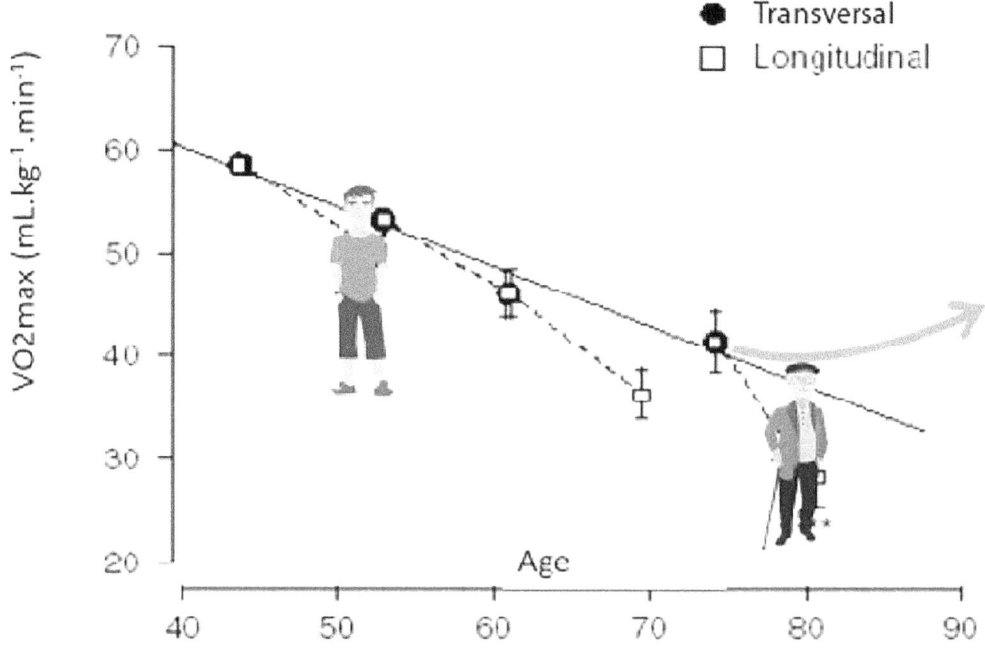

Figure 34. The decrease in VO2 max with age in males. The green arrow represents the effects of acceleration training in elderly males.

Sarcopenia – loss of muscle mass with age

Functional centenarians represent an impressive example of successful healthy aging. Aging is a continuum of biological processes, characterized by progressive adaptations heavily influenced by genetic and physiological factors. However, even in these truly unique individuals, declining lung function and sarcopenia (loss of muscle) lead to a progressive fall in strength and reduced exercise capacity. The limitation in mobility can initiate a vicious decline in physical function and health. Recent studies have shed some light on this multi-factorial decline in function associated with aging and the decisive role that diet and exercise play in the elderly. Controlling sarcopenia is especially crucial in maintaining independence and function in centenarians.

Quick facts about sarcopenia

- Sarcopenia can start as early as age 30
- 100 percent of centenarians have sarcopenia

- Only 10 percent of centenarians are physically independent. Meaning they can function alone in their own homes.

No need to wait for more studies, the funding is sparse for this type of research.

Low muscle mass and strength are independently and significantly associated with an increase of all-cause mortality among U.S. older adults regardless of muscle mass, metabolic syndrome risk factors, sedentary time, or leisure-time physical activity. Similarly, people with higher cholesterol levels are also less likely to die (Tuikkala, 2010). Rather than worrying about weight or body mass index, we should be focusing more on maintaining muscle mass. Muscle physiology experts recommend that protein intake be increased as we age. A sedentary lifestyle and lack of exercise is a significant risk factor for sarcopenia. Muscle fiber numbers begin to decrease around 40 – 50 years of age. The decline in muscle fiber and strength is more pronounced in patients with sedentary lifestyles than patients who work out. Even professional athletes such as marathon runners and weightlifters show a gradual, albeit slower decline in their speed and strength with aging.

Age-related decreases in hormone concentrations, testosterone, thyroid hormone, and insulin-like growth factor, lead to a loss of muscle mass and strength. Extreme muscle loss often results from a combination of diminishing hormonal anabolic signals and inflammation. A decrease in the body's ability to synthesize protein, coupled with an inadequate intake of calories and quality protein to sustain muscle mass, is common in sarcopenia. Oxidized muscle proteins increase with age and lead to a buildup of what are called cross-linked proteins. These proteins are not easily removed (via the proteolysis system). This leads to an accumulation of non-contractile, dysfunctional protein in skeletal muscles, and another reason muscle strength decreases in sarcopenia. This model may change as the body becomes less insulin resistant, and protein optimization takes place. Evolutionary theories implicate sedentary behavior and the failure of the human body to maintain muscle mass and function with aging. This hypothesis suggests that genes suited for high levels of obligatory muscular effort, i.e., running from tigers, were required for survival in the

> late Paleolithic era. High levels of lifelong sedentary behavior characterize our modern lifestyle—a fancy way of saying use or lose it.
>
> Sarcopenic Obesity is a medical condition in which low lean body mass is combined with high-fat mass. It is associated with impaired functional capacity, disability, metabolic complications, and increased mortality. Low muscle mass, along with high-fat mass, is also characteristic of the aging process. Likewise, we know that obesity greatly increases the chance of death. Many studies that investigate how obesity and weight affect the risk of death look only at BMI. But it should be noted there is no gold-standard measure of body composition, several studies have addressed this question using different measurement techniques and have obtained different results. It has long been thought that age-related weight loss and a loss of muscle mass were mostly responsible for muscle weakness in older people. However, studies in patients with Sarcopenic Obesity reveal that changes in muscle composition are also significant. Marbling or fat infiltration into muscle lowers muscle quality and work performance.

We recently demonstrated that an increase in VO2 max from 30 – 40 is possible in a one-hundred-five-year-old male cyclist trained by focusing on the variation of the cadence rate between 70 – 90 revolutions per minute (Billat 2017). Also, recall the Irish fifty-nine-year-old marathoner with a VO2 max of 69.5 ml/kg/min. Our results support the previous high-intensity interval training (HIIT) results, with exercise sessions of fifteen 30-second periods, each at 90 – 95 percent of maximum heart rate, which can improve VO2 max in a younger population (Serna 2016). However, HIIT training is likely too painful for the body beyond 50 or 60 years of age. Research studies using a modified HIIT protocol in humans has shown that a series of 1 to 9 repetitions of 30 seconds at maximum speed with a long recovery (6 minutes), three times a week, resulted in a 40 percent reduction in mileage and increases the muscle's ability to resist fatigue. Also, these types of training sessions increase the rate of enzymes promoting the catabolism of glucose and optimizing the rate of lactate transporters for the removal of lactate (Puype 2013).

Choosing the strategy of speed variation training is challenging to maintain for beginners or even advanced non-professional runners. There are many beneficial effects on the metabolic regulators of anaerobic glycolysis and the muscle (both skeletal and cardiac) that optimize the regulation of calcium and proteins, which promote the cellular transport of sodium, potassium, chlorine (anti-cramp factors). Performance improves with accelerated-based training sessions (Easy, Medium, and Hard), resulting in reduced mileage and increases both oxidative and non-oxidative capabilities.

ADDING LIFE TO LIFE. TEDX TALK BY DR. BILLAT

Using acceleration and deceleration during training aims to augment well-being and performance to earn "miles" of life! Ajouter de la vie a la vie (Adding life to life) is the title of a TEDx conference that Dr. Billat had the pleasure of giving at the Lille CNAM in 2016 (in French, see youtube.com).

CHAPTER 13 SUMMARY

CONCEPT: The word "qualitative training" means to use your senses, run by feel, don't try to put numbers on it. By understanding and practicing minimalistic qualitative training, you will arrive at a place where you will instinctively train without putting undue stress on the body and run into your later years. We all desire to be able to run and train into our later years, but with age, we lose several physiologic mechanisms. For example, we lose the ability to recover our muscles like when we were in our 20's. One of the first things humans lose with age is quick muscle control. This is due to nervous system changes in the myelin sheaths surrounding the axons are gradually degraded and reduced—our brain chemistry changes with age. For example, the production of certain neurotransmitters (the chemical molecules that transmit messages from one neuron to another) declines with age. Qualitative training based on accelerations and decelerations helps curb the decrease in strength and muscle mass during aging.

APPLICATION: Training with a good cadence is the main goal as we age. This decrease of the nerve firing rate is the main cause of power loss in our running speeds; an excellent example is that it becomes difficult to have a high cadence (>150 – 160) or be able to sprint over 15 mph (25 kph). By integrating accelerations of 10 seconds, starting from a zone of average speed and repeating them 10 times every 3 minutes, for example, will help to avoid musculoskeletal injuries and cardiovascular stress.

CHAPTER 14

LISTEN TO YOUR BODY

Today, it sounds strange to listen to your feelings while running a marathon. With the plethora of wearable devices available nowadays, we are conditioned to run according to a digital display instead of running to how we feel. Acceleration-based training is about listening to your feelings while simultaneously optimizing your performance. As we have already pointed out, humans run instinctively by varying the pace and discern the difference between easy, moderate, and hard. Our natural ability to regulate our accelerations gives us the ability to manage our energy resources during a marathon. It takes practice to develop the perceptions necessary for perfect regulation of the physiologic loads we place on our bodies to manage our energy resources better. By learning to manage our energies, we can attain the possibility of achieving our best results.

Acceleration-based training naturally develops our ability to vary the running speed. By increasing the acuity of our racing sensations, you will learn to adjust your physiological load naturally. Combine this with increased power, and you will solicit your true VO2 max. Imagine running without being polluted by a cognitive control that consists of running while scanning the heart rate-GPS watch. Admittingly, the new technologies are useful for validating specific physiologic parameters. Our biofeedback can be natural from devices. However, we lose it when we want to control everything consciously, or worse. We become so exhausted that we no longer feel connected to our bodies. How many times have we had the uncomfortable feeling of not being able to control our legs? Lack of sleep, stress, glycogen depletion, overtraining, and pain affects us more than we know.

Having proper energy resource management by varying your speed will save time and let you recover while running. But for this to work, a realistic estimate of our physiological load must be chosen to run at a compatible speed variation. Indeed, we have innate warning mechanisms that prevent us from subjecting our body to rigorous efforts that are incompatible with our homeostasis. The French physiologist, Claude Bernard, developed the theory of homeostasis, which maintains the natural balance of the internal environment. Training consists of safely pushing our limits, stimulating physiological adaptations, and not forcing yourself to overcome them. An excellent example of the latter is that those who use performance-enhancing drugs can no longer feel their natural sensations. The subjective approach of estimating the difficulty of an exercise is called the "Rate of Perceived Exertion" or RPE, which was developed by Borg in the 1970s (Figure 35). Assuming the perception of the difficulty of exercise is proportional to heart rate and blood lactate, Borg developed a scale that corresponds to heart rate ranging from 6 to 20. To use the Borg scale, an athlete would choose the difficulty perceived from an exercise and multiply the index of the scale by 10, to find its heart rate value in beats per minute (bpm).

In theory, RPE is considered a psycho-physiological construct affected by both physiological and psychological variables (Eston 2012). For example, changes in heart rate, oxygen uptake, muscle glycogen levels, and concentrations of brain neurotransmitters such as dopamine may affect RPE responses to exercise (St Clair Gibson 2001).

Changes in emotions also influence both the RPE and exercise performance (Baronet 2011). It has been suggested that RPE is a robust variable that indicates the subjective tolerance of the individual to exercise at a given intensity (Hampson 2001). RPE has also recently been used to estimate steady-state lactate formation while running at a constant pace. An associated workload corresponding to an RPE rating of 13 could estimate the exercise intensity corresponding to maximum steady-state lactate. However, it is more a question of looking at RPE and a steady-state zone of lactate while varying the speed. A physiological examination testing the different metabolisms (Molinari 2018) shows that to stay in a perceived perception zone as being "average" (corresponding to an RPE of 13 – 14), the runner needs to follow a variation of speed in successive waves of short durations (less than 1 minute).

Rating	Descriptor
6	No exertion at all
7	Extremely light
8	
9	Very light
10	
11	Light
12	
13	Somewhat hard
14	
15	Hard (heavy)
16	
17	Very Hard
18	
19	Extremely hard

Figure 35. Fatigue perception scale: RPE ("Ratings of Perceived Exertion" How do you perceive the effort? (Borg, 1970).

At BillaTraining.com, we only use five areas of perception of the Borg scale to correlate physiological load. The Borg scale can be oversensitive at times, and there may be a problem of understanding the nuances of "extremely, very, slightly, etc." An excellent example of perceived exertion that every runner has experienced is the intensity at which it is no longer possible to speak and increased respiratory rate. This constitutes a threshold of perceived exertion which is well correlated with the lowering of blood-muscle pH which causes a heaviness in the legs and appear before hyperventilation.

The length of a race often dictates what we will feel at a certain distance or time. For example, during a half or full marathon, we will adjust our pace according to the physiological stresses that we feel at specific points in the race. If we anticipate our legs will feel weak around the halfway point, we will slow our pace, hoping to avoid the catastrophe of bonking. Some runners prefer to use time and other distance. Often, elite runners prefer time or distance markers every four minutes or every kilometer. Using the time markers relative to distance allows us to forget about the speed (remember that the distance is the product of the speed and time).

Similarly, some runners run according to absolute speed (km/hr) or relative (%MAS) or pace. This can lead to better energy management by finding a variation of the comfortable pace that is acquired with experience. If you force yourself to run at a constant speed and ignoring your sensations, the marathon will likely not end well. During a race, using the Borg scale is too difficult to adjust your pace according to your perceived exertion. Again, the reason why we need to keep it simple and use the five levels of perception:

- **Easy**
- **Medium**
- **Hard**
- **Very Hard**
- **Sprinting**

These were the perceived exertion scales that came before the Borg scale. We even tested these five levels of perceived exertion with 10-year-old children. We had them follow a Rabit® test (Figure 35), and they were able to distinguish the intensities by simply following instructions. In fact, in the adults we tested, the "easy" pace corresponded to 65 percent of the "very hard" speed; "average" pace corresponded to 80 percent of the "very hard" speed and the very hard speed correlated to about 90 percent of the "very hard" speed, and finally sprinting (6 seconds) corresponded to 120 percent of the "very hard."

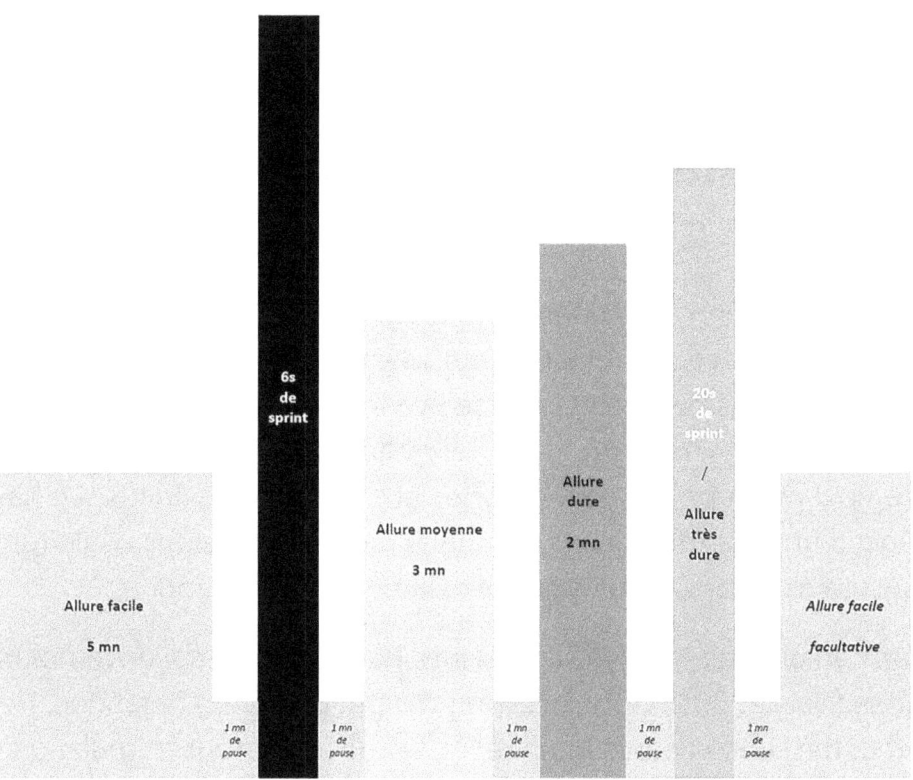

Figure 36. Rabit® test protocol for children under 16 years of age. Allure facile = Easy Pace, Allure Moyen = Medium Pace, Allure Dure = Hard Pace, Allure Très Dure = Very Hard Pace, Pause = Rest.

We believe that the five levels of perceived exertion are natural and incredibly easy to follow. We were able to show that 3rd-grade children were perfectly able to distinguish different running paces when instructed using the different levels of exertion. Even more, the gaits for each level are different. The heart rate remains at steady state within the perceived intensity levels despite the change in speed (or precisely because of this spontaneous speed variation). The 10-year-olds are already able to interpret a verbal command of intensity that was well formulated by the physical education teacher. Another interesting study done twenty years ago demonstrated that a runner could accurately estimate the time he can hold at a constant speed (Garcin 1999). This suggests that during a free-running race, the runner constantly manages his speed variation according to the time he or she thinks he can hold at a given speed. Logically, a runner cannot sustain a speed higher than his/her comfort zone speed. An Estimate Time Limit (ETL) scale was validated using a constant speed model in field studies. But this is yet to be worked out in a freely managed race model in terms of speed versus target race distance.

HOW THE BRAIN AFFECTS YOUR POWER OUTPUT DURING RUNNING

With all this discussion about how to judge your level of exercise through the Borg scale and RPE, we should talk about why the brain is so important to running a marathon. As discussed, we use five levels of RPE in our BillaTraining.com programs: easy, medium, hard, very hard, and sprinting. The brain can regulate how much power your muscles put out while running. We have all experienced unpleasant feelings of fatigue and even illusions while running. This may seem obvious, but it is useful to know why this happens.

South African physiologist Tim Noakes introduced the central governor model of exercise (Noakes 2011) for explaining the phenomenon of fatigue. He proposed that the subconscious brain regulates power output (stimulation strategy) by modulating muscle motor unit recruitment to preserve homeostasis and prevent catastrophic physiological failures such as severe muscle rigor and cell death. In this model, the word fatigue is redefined. Instead of the decline in the ability to produce strength and power from your muscles, it is more about the neural fatigue affecting sensations and emotions. The brain uses unpleasant sensations of fatigue to ensure that the exercise intensity remains within a person's physiologic capacity. Thus, this model predicts that your best performances are going to be achieved by controlling the progression of these illusory symptoms during exercise.

While the central governor model is useful for explaining brain regulation of exercise, a variety of peripheral factors other than hypoxia, hydration, temperature, lactate, and muscle acidosis are known to compromise strength and muscle power. Instead, it is suggested that the concept of task dependence, in which the mechanisms of fatigue vary according to the specific exercise stressor, is a better explanation and defensible model of fatigue. This model includes both central and peripheral aspects contributions to fatigue, and the relative importance of each probably varies with the type of exercise. The fatigue model of the central governor postulates:

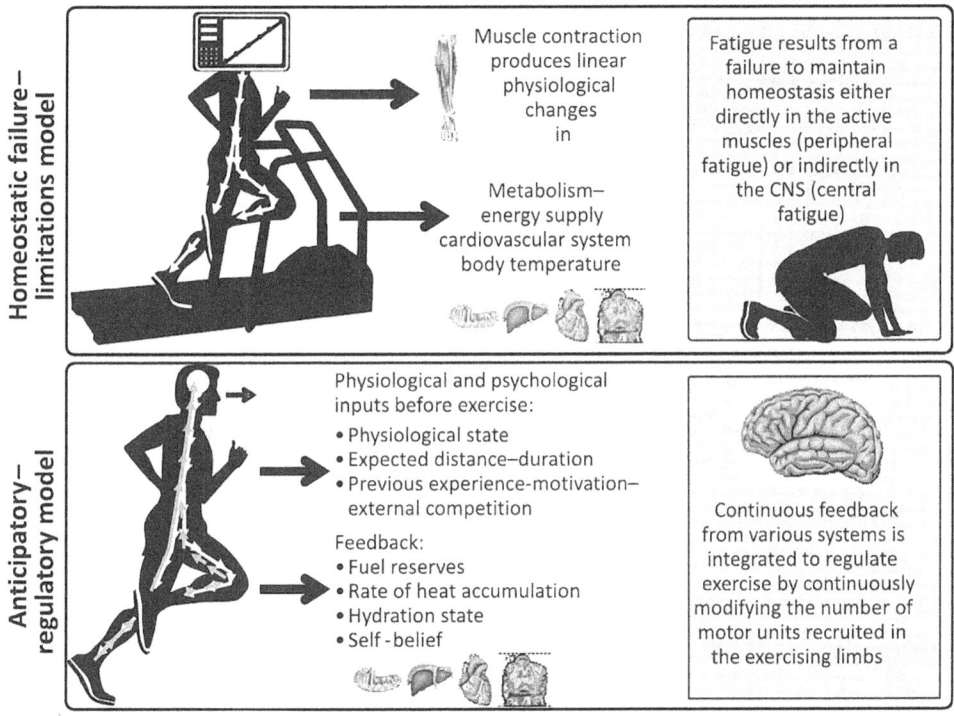

Figure 37. Theory of pace control and the Central Governor theory (Noakes 2011).

"The brain regulates the performance of exercise by the recruitment of motor units, in particular in conjunction with inhibitory signals mediated by unpleasant sensations of fatigue."

In this model, the brain adjusts motor unit recruitment to avoid "catastrophic system failure" and fatigue is redefined from a physical manifestation as a decrease in the capacity to produce force at a given sensation/emotion for a given condition.

The central governor theory does not work for exercises such as the marathon or a 30-second sprint at full speed. Numerous studies show that exercise and performance can be limited centrally by the recruitment of the neural units (central fatigue of cerebral origin), but also by the loss of contractile performance of the skeletal muscle itself. If you continue to run at the same speeds, you, therefore, put the same tension and length on the muscle fibers. Also, the central governor model still needs to incorporate known fatigue modulation of muscle activation into the spinal cord. It proposes that the brain plans an action in its subconscious before an exercise and regulates motor unit recruitment continuously during exercise using feelings of exhaustion, such as the Borg scale. It should be noted that the maximum steady-state velocity of blood lactate corresponds to an RPE of 14 ± 2, depending on the individual.

RPE is also dependent on the education and social position of the person. Among the many runners who come to us to get back into shape or prepare for a sporting event, we have found that women CEO's and executives or those who have an education that emphasized hard work and difficulties can reach their ventilatory threshold and VO2 max at a declared RPE of 10 – 13. Indeed, it is impossible to know if they are holding back or intentionally pushing themselves past their thresholds. In any case, these women often feel that they have not given their maximum and are dissatisfied with their performance. Male executives and CEOs, on the other hand, often declare an RPE close to 20, even when they are not truly at the end of their effort, at least in terms of reaching the maximum oxygen consumption or heart rate. They often do not reach 90 percent of their theoretical maximal heart rate (210 - 0.65 × age), and blood lactate greater than 8 mmol/L of blood. Despite our observations, nothing has been truly demonstrated in this area despite a mountain of publications on the subject. The protocols being designed for such studies are far from ideal and often force them to undergo "disappointments" on their running time or use a distorted clock. These studies ignore the true motivation that goes into an actual race.

It is especially important to understand the "feelings" that arise while you are training or racing. We do not attempt to separate pacing studies from those on the notion of "central governor theory" (figure 36) as they often lead into inutile debates. These arguments are complex and include neurophysiology, mathematics, physiology, and even cognitive psychology to understand better this notion of "feeling" (Damasio 2013). Thus, the latter manages to make a sketch, a kind of thought experiment, as to the link between homeostasis, entropy, and feeling. There is consensus that for low intensities (inducing a minimum of discomfort for RPE <11-12), the brain can regulate muscle activity automatically without thinking about it. While beyond an RPE of 15 (intensity perceived as hard), we are in a state of active vigilance. Vigilance is defined as the state of readiness to detect.

MIND GAMES

Many scientists have attempted to explain how the mind controls the body during exercise. The Explanatory Theory of Pace Control states that homeostasis controls the recruitment of muscular motor fibers. The anticipatory model and feedback loop that adds a dimension of strategic anticipation as a function of the anticipation of the runner as to his sensations as a function of time and distance that will act as a comparator and will modulate his pace depending on the possible difference between what was expected and what is perceived (Noakes 2011). We react to discrete changes occurring at varying intervals within the environment. In the race, beyond a certain difficulty of effort, we feel the effects and too much vigilance will cause us to slow down. Some runners like to say that they have the feeling of "dropping their brains" to avoid stopping. Others may say they are "running out of their head." Therefore, it is necessary to mix resilience and dare to have the curiosity to continue your accelerations or at least maintain the speed a little longer. By thinking this way, you will not run too slow!

Modern neuroscience only offers the model of the Bayesian brain, which dares to make bets and anticipatory decisions. This is where the master runner takes his revenge by sorting out the bet, acts on the critical sensations, and leaves the insignificant ones aside. As in life, we can discern what is important. We have a saying in French, *we keep our friends, and we set aside the donkey skins and useless objects*. The spirit of the marathon is the symbol of avoiding the rat race. We adopt a minimalist training using our sensations in terms of the acceleration's dosage, resulting in positive and negative speed variations. The result should be a speed variation that results in the synchronicity of our metabolism.

We can summarize human intentionality from a Bayesian perspective. After selecting the most likely interpretation of sensory inputs by Bayesian processing of these inputs, the brain uses the stored-data directory that resembles the current situation. This interpretation is transmitted to the decision centers, compared to the repertoire of possible actions. These actions are dependent on the memory of racing experiences. The final decision depends on the gain that can be expected (and pain relief is part of that gain) for each possible action (Ernst and Bültoff 2004). This is how artificial intelligence can be applied to this probabilistic approach of the brain to study the probability of accelerating positively, negatively, or nil, depending on the cost functions in relation to the gain. Imagine having to beat your avatar in a video game where it would be a matter of choosing speed variations, a new speed signature that would deceive this artificial intelligence. In this sense, our brains are not robots, and we naturally prefer an unbridled race! Beyond the analysis of the curves of speed and acceleration, it would be interesting to analyze the runner's language. It will be a question of being able to evaluate the form of a person who has characteristic, recurring words, which could be his true linguistic signature to express his perception of the race. Training can then be readjusted session by session accordingly to optimize performance. We always return to the question of the liberation of the race and our thoughts.

To achieve the most out of these four discoveries, you must trust and learn to connect with yourself. To free your neurons from the old paradigms, we will arm ourselves with the current training concepts and the valuable experience of the sage coaches that know how to keep us healthy. Dr. Billat made her revolution in the field of running. It took three decades to explore the limits of the notions of MAS, VO2 max, aerobic thresholds, critical speed, and endurance.

CHAPTER 14 SUMMARY

CONCEPT: Acceleration based training is about listening to your feelings and, at the same time, optimizing your performance. Humans run instinctively by varying the pace and can easily discern the difference between easy, medium, and hard. Our natural ability to regulate our accelerations is what gives us the ability to manage our energy resources during a marathon. It takes practice to develop the perceptions necessary for perfect regulation of the physiologic loads we place on our bodies resulting in better energy management. By learning to manage our energies, we can attain the possibility of achieving our best results. Acceleration based training naturally develops our ability to vary the speed. By increasing the acuity of our racing sensations, you will learn to adjust your physiological load naturally. Combine this with increased power, and you will solicit your true VO2 max. And all this without being polluted by a cognitive control that consists of running while scanning the GPS watch.

APPLICATION: Today, it sounds strange listening to your feelings while running a marathon. With the plethora of wearable devices available nowadays, we are conditioned to run according to a digital display instead of running to how we feel. Admittingly, the new technologies are useful for validating certain physiologic parameters. Attempt to optimize your biofeedback naturally, even if you are using a device. However, we lose it when we want to control everything consciously or when we are concerned about our problems or worse, so exhausted that we no longer feel connected to our bodies. Run without looking at the GPS-watch and see how close you can come to run the pace you feel naturally.

CHAPTER 15

THE BILLATRAINING PROGRAM

The BillaTraining.com method is based on two main principles:

- Respect your running sensations.
- Optimize the training load for better recovery and fewer injuries.

Achieving these principles gives you the ability to understand your sensations while training and racing accurately. This allows you to avoid over and undertraining and maximize the effectiveness of your training. Increasing your power reserve is essential to accomplish all of this. We will teach you how to validate your running sensations with the simple analysis of your GPS-watch curves. We hope to give you the possibility of running a race (with or without a number) and having the impression of trotting or galloping! No animal on earth runs at a constant pace. The way horses and dogs run is a constant inspiration, and running brings us closer to them.

Every athlete in the BillaTraining.com program undergoes an energy audit stage with the Rabit® test to define your energy profile. From this new vision of the marathon and the four fundamentals that we have described in the first chapter, we will individualize your training program. Discovering your true "speed signature" is defined as your optimal variation of speed. Running according to your speed signature is the variation of pace, allowing you to optimize the synchronization of your "aerobic-anaerobic hybrid engine."

The BillaTraining.com method works in 3 steps:

1. The energy audit with the Rabit® test

2. Build a training program according to your energy profile

3. Developing your speed signature for your event.

THE ENERGY AUDIT

The energy audit defines your physiological characteristics in response to the Rabit® test. Every aspect of your running performance will be highlighted by the analysis of the Rabit® test and without focusing on VO2 max. Remember that VO2 max is an artifact, i.e., the maximum oxygen consumption for a single test, a precise protocol resulting from the traditional VAMEVAL test. We like to refer to a VO2 max test as the "corridor of the little death." The last two minutes of a VO2 test are fateful since the only outcome is complete physical and mental exhaustion; we do not focus on this in the BillaTraining.com method. The Rabit® test allows you to know your energy profile to better train and run. By validating your effort with your sensations, you will avoid constant pace running. You will refine your ability to accelerate and decelerate momentarily, which is the key to letting your "motor" recover. By eliminating the lactate produced, you will better recharge your creatine phosphate and better preserve intramuscular glycogen.

THE RABIT® TEST

The Rabit® test protocol is a test based on your sensations, permitting you to push the limits and allowing you to vary the speed and avoiding running at a constant pace. The main objective of the Rabit® is to build the athlete's energy profile according to the four performance factors: Force-speed or power, Tolerance to acidosis, Perception of the physiological load, and Cardiovascular efficiency. To develop an indvidualized training program that develops all of the energy metabolisms, the www.BillaTraining.com method has built and validated the Rabit® test (Molinari 2018). The test consists of linking various instructions based on the athlete's perception. The test is broken down into several stages, with a one-minute recovery between each stage (in blue). Determining your energetic profile using the Rabit® test consists of running less than thirty minutes with a simple set of perceived intensities (Easy, Medium,

Hard, Very hard, Sprint). The recovery minute is a phase where the runner walks or jogs slowly.

The Rabit® Test:

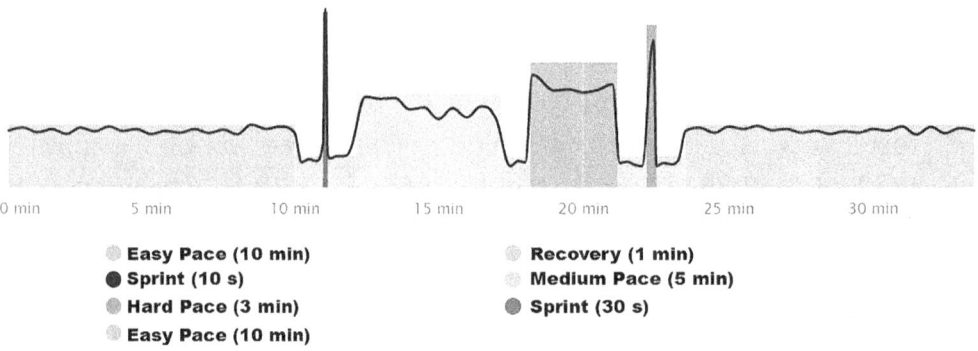

- Easy Pace (10 min)
- Sprint (10 s)
- Hard Pace (3 min)
- Easy Pace (10 min)
- Recovery (1 min)
- Medium Pace (5 min)
- Sprint (30 s)

- 10 minutes at a pace felt as being "Easy" (in green), then walk/jog for 1 minute (in blue)

- A short sprint of 10 seconds (in black), then walk/jog for 1 minute (in blue)

- 5 minutes at pace felt as "Medium" (in orange), then walk/jog for 1 minute (in blue)

- 3 minutes at a pace felt as being "difficult or hard" (in red), then walk/jog for 1 minute (in blue)

- A 30-second sprint (in gray), then walk/jog for 1 minute (in blue)

- 5 to 10 minutes at a pace felt to be "Easy" (in green)

VALIDATION OF THE RABIT® TEST

The Rabit® test allows us to produce a profile of a runners' entire metabolism and speed spectrum. The Rabit® test also makes it possible to discover the range of perceived speeds. Similarly, the less stressful Rabit® test makes it possible to measure VO2 max within five percent of actual values. The differences are due to the biological variability and are inherent in measuring respiratory gas exchanges, especially in the field. It is important to note that the runners who had never done the Rabit® test were perfectly able to distinguish the different phases. We have excellent research showing that the Rabit® test is reproducible. A new way to run the marathon is discovered: the physiological approach to running a marathon under the prism of sensation and variable speeds rather than that of treadmill tests with imposed constant speeds. However, some runners have difficulty distinguishing an average speed from a hard speed or an easy speed from an average speed. Self-evaluation of your energy profile after your Rabit® test is done with a simple algorithm-free approach. While the Rabit® test algorithm is proprietary, you can apply this self-assessment from the questionnaire for each factor on our website, and we will give you access to many useful workouts. Knowing these intensities will make it possible to know your energy profile, individualize your training program, and your speed signature. Remember that the speed signature is the speed variation that allows you to get the fastest time possible, given your current fitness level. The essential physical qualities for running fast, long with ease and pleasure are Power, Tolerance to Acidosis, Cardiac Efficiency, and Perception of physiological effort.

THE ENERGY RADAR

At BillaTraining.com, we use the energy radar to individualize and quantify the four pillars of marathon performance. To create the energy radar the runner must score their Force, Perception, Cardiac Efficiency, and Tolerance to Acidosis. To create an accurate energy radar, it is best to work with a knowledgeable coach and have experience with these types of assessments.

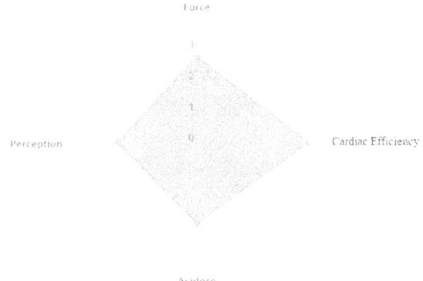

Figure 38. This runner's energy radar shows that he has a large cardiovascular capacity, which is noted by the fact that he attained a heart rate well past his predicted heart rate.

FORCE-SPEED (F)

The power reserve (speed) is something that we have emphasized throughout this book and is among the most limiting factors in marathon running and is the key to success! The BillaTraining.com training program is designed to help you accomplish your marathon transformation based on the power gain and, therefore, the speed reserve to be more comfortable at a given pace. For example, a pace of 8 min/mile (5 min/km) will appear "easy" whereas it would have seemed "average" to you with a classic training based on constant paced volume and tempo training. We must look at the quality of the power-speed relationship to consider improving your marathon record. This first item of your energy profile is the most limiting. Therefore, it is necessary to increase your maximum power (best understood as the product of strength and speed). We must have a speed reserve between a comfortable speed (easy) and a maximum speed (sprint). It is necessary to increase the maximum stride power and, therefore, the strength and frequency (velocity) at high speed. The maximum oxygen consumption, which has been considered for more than a century as the main factor of performance, can only be achieved if we can produce enough power. How many runners tell you that they cannot raise their heart rate? A maximum heart rate cannot be obtained without enough stimulation at a neuromuscular level. Without power, we cannot solicit our VO2 max.

On the other hand, our power reserve runs over long distances, allowing us to vary the speed so that we can use all our energy metabolisms in a synchronized manner (aerobic and anaerobic). Varying the speed and therefore, the length of shortening of the muscle fibers is essential to efficiency. Having muscular strength avoids "pushing you into the ground" at the thirtieth km. Finally, this avoids having to double your support time to maintain your speed with the same impulse (Pulse = Force × ground support time). Strength is, therefore a critical factor in energy efficiency.

TOLERANCE TO ACIDOSIS (A)

A common limiting factor in marathoners is tolerance to acidosis. Having a good tolerance to acidosis for high power energy storage is important. Certainly, the possibility of storing energy in the form of lactate is a primal quality of being human. Lactate recycling is a result of varying the pace along with an adequate speed reserve. Lactate is used in the acceleration phases. In addition, to effectively eliminate the muscle acidosis, you must be able to perform maximum efforts (30 seconds to 3 minutes) to reach the maximum power engine (VO2 max) to eliminate acidosis.

CARDIAC EFFICACY (C)

The third limiting factor in energy performance is cardiac efficiency. Remember, the heart pumps nearly 2000 gallons per day (7,500 liters)! Your heart muscle must be able to eject a large volume of blood in a short time and at a high rate and be efficient at sub-maximum speeds to preserve its oxygen consumption. The blood flow (which is the product of the heart rate and the stroke volume) must provide enough oxygen to the tissues to increase the running speed. The oxygen consumption of the myocardium (MVO2) is proportional to the square of the heart rate. As soon as your heart rate increases, it increases the cardiac output but also the MVO2. With proper training, your heart rate will lower at a given speed and increase your maximum heart rate for increased blood flow and oxygen consumption to go faster and longer.

PERCEPTION OF EXERCISE INTENSITY (P)

Perception is everything. What you perceive while running is your "connection" to your relative intensity level (percent V02 max).

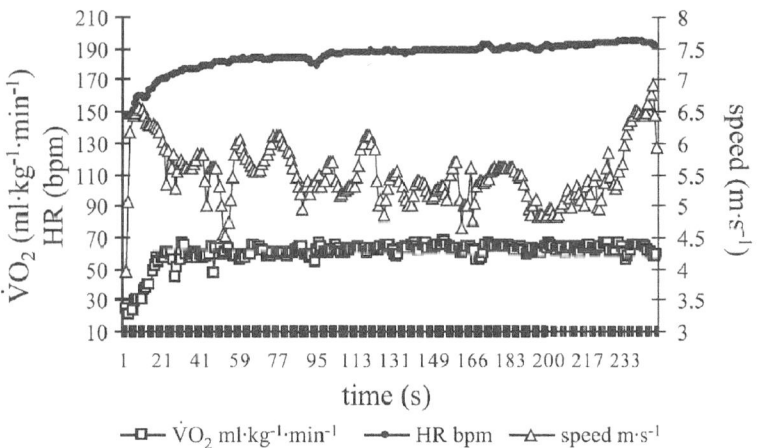

Figure 39. 1500-m race in competition. The runner varies his speed from 4.5 – 7 m/s (17 – 25 km/hr) while VO2 max caps and the heart rate (HR) increase (Billat 2009).

Your perception is about maintaining a stable physiological state at different levels (easy, medium, hard). By varying running speeds, we can maintain the maximum oxygen consumption longer while running at intensities considered "hard" near VO2 max. This is difficult to emulate on a treadmill or progressive incremental triangular tests where the runner cannot recover by slowing down. Remember, we have shown that reducing the speed and increasing it again allows a further increase in VO2 as well as the plateau duration to VO2 max (Petot 2012). Moreover, during a 1500-m race, the runners had a long plateau of VO2 max at speed superior to baseline MAS (Figure 40). At speed "very hard," we are running all out. Understand that the real value of the Rabit® test lies in the fact that the runner will give free rein to his/her sensations and what is understood to be a set of "easy, medium and hard" feelings. This is different than the classical method of managing short extended sprints of 30 seconds at maximum speed.

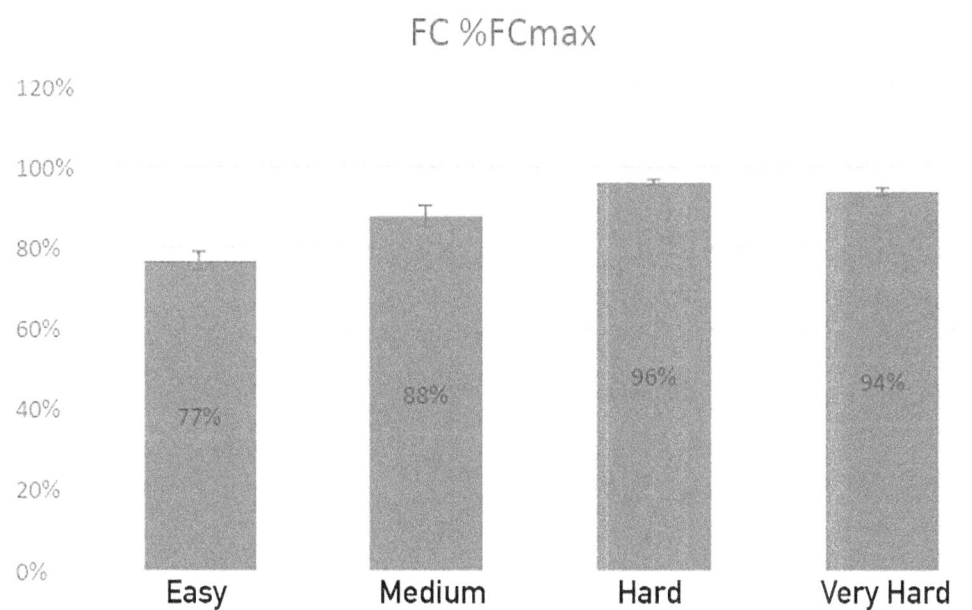

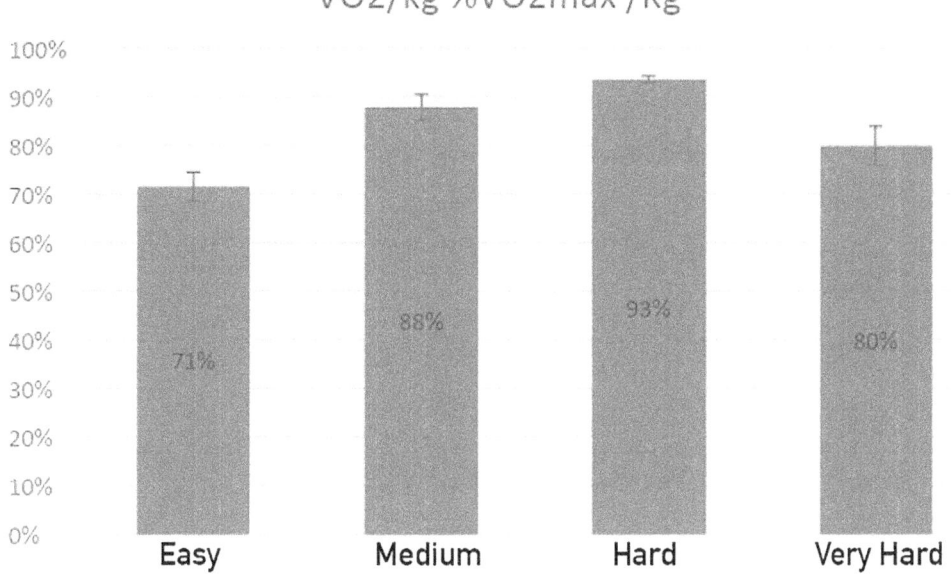

Figures 40. Positioning of the perceived velocities in terms of %VO2 max and %HR max during a Rabit® test on runners of all levels.

We can see in figure 40 that we can perfectly perceive the different intensity levels relative to VO2 max, maximum heart rate (HR max), speed, and reproducibility (Molinari 2018). We have strongly emphasized the need to have a perception of your physiological state to be able to accelerate or deaccelerate at any time while running subconsciously. Do not forget that this "choice" is made at small time intervals of 4 seconds; which is the period of uncertainty for which the brain does not perceive sensory signals (tension, length of muscle, body temperature, acidosis, blood pressure in O2 and CO2, nociceptive pain by type III and IV sensory fibers, hyperventilation). But to increase this sensitivity of your physiological state, you must increase the amplitude of power to figure out your "potentiometer" and relative power. For that, you must increase your power reserve; that is why we suggest you include it in your energy audit because it is one of the four pillars of your profile to build your personalized training.

POWER AND EXPLOSIVENESS

Remember that power is the product of force and speed, and that as we age, we lose more speed than strength. Here's an interesting anecdote: a 2-year-old has the same relative strength as a young adult. After 50 years of age, we have more difficulty turning the legs over and have an increased stride frequency, limiting our speed gain beyond 12 mph or 20 kph. Do not take the lead with cadence (frequency) trying to control it, but it can be instructive to evaluate your neuromuscular fatigue and your power in training and racing. Quite often, when we are fatigued (work, stress, jet lag), we are unable to control our cadence, and this results in a loss of power. Learn to stay warm under the covers one Sunday morning per month, for example. Recovery is part of training as well.

How Muscles Develop Power

A muscle develops its power according to the laws of the length-tension relationship and the force-velocity relationship. In practical terms, it is not because you can squat a heavyweight that allows you to accelerate up a hill at a faster rate. The primary determinant of this mechanical loading in the running is the force-velocity relationship. However, the length-tension relationship can also affect, and it explains why full ranges of motion (long strides) and eccentric training produce the results. The classic example of an eccentric exercise quadriceps is walking downstairs or running downhill.

In humans, hypertrophy (an increase in the size of a whole muscle) is almost entirely the result of single muscle fibers increasing in volume. This usually occurs due to an increase in muscle fiber diameter, but also happens because of increases in muscle fiber length. While increases in the number of muscle fibers happen in rodents, the same results have never been duplicated in humans. Moreover, bodybuilders seem to have approximately the same number of muscle fibers in a muscle as untrained individuals, despite having much larger muscles. The force produced by any given muscle fiber during a muscular contraction (and therefore the degree of mechanical loading that it experiences) is primarily determined by whether the muscle fiber is activated and the speed at which the muscle fiber shortens due to the force-velocity relationship. Again, remember that the main determinant of the mechanical loading experienced by active muscle fibers in a muscular contraction is the force-velocity relationship.

The technical capacity of applying force (or mechanical efficiency) during the sprint can be quantified at each step by calculating the ratio of the horizontal and ground reaction forces (GRF). If we look at the entire phase of rate acceleration (RA), which decreases linearly as speed increases, the rate acceleration, describes the ability to maintain a forward horizontal orientation of the resulting GRF vector despite an increase in velocity. What is important here is the concept of strength-endurance and its relation to the forces generated with each step. To detect a state of fatigue racing with tools such as a heart rate GPS-watch unit, we can look for a decrease in cadence and an increase in ground contact time. The best way to avoid neuromuscular fatigue is, therefore:

1. Increase your maximum power reserve to run at a lower percentage of that power for the same race speed. Keep in mind that the sprint speed that corresponds to the runner's MAS gives a zone, a physiological and perceptual state, rather than a precise speed. Those "precise speeds" are instead found on the treadmill tests of an artificial triangular protocol (VAMEVAL) that leads to exhaustion without the ability to recover for better acceleration.

2. Vary the speed during training and running to release the muscles, never allowing the same muscle length and muscle tension.

CARDIAC EFFICIENCY (CARDIO)

The actual maximum heart rate (HR max) of the sprint speed must be higher than 90 percent of your theoretical maximum heart rate = 210 - 0.65 × age (number of years). After running hard for 3 minutes and one minute of recovery, you must go back to less than 80 percent of your max HR. After one minute of recovery after the sprint, your HR should return to less than 80 percent of the sprint max HR.

Remember that cardiac efficiency is vital for many things, such as bringing oxygen and lactate to the muscles. The oxygen consumption depends on the cardiac output, and blood ejected from the heart with each heartbeat. Cardiac output is the product of the volume of blood ejected at each emptying of your left ventricle (the volume of systolic ejection SEV) multiplied by the heart rate. We must strive for the highest HR max possible despite aging. Aging causes us to lose 0.65 beats per year according to the theoretical equation based on statistics:

$$\text{Theoretical HR max} = 210 - 0.65 \times \text{age in number of years.}$$

Equation 220 - age (years) is less accurate since it lowers the HR one beat per year. A good example is our cyclist 106-year-old, Robert Marchand. Theoretically, he should have had a HR max equal to 220 - 103 = 117 bpm. But he achieved an HR max of 156 bpm!

The heart is an efficient consumer of lactate. Recycling lactic acid is particularly important for our purposes since the heart (muscle) is a consumer of lactate for its contractions. In a marathon, the heart contracts about 30,000 times in 3 hours, assuming an average HR of 160 bpm. Because the heart cons of consumes a lot of oxygen, especially with high cardiac output, recovery is more efficient with a full heart that is adequately hydrated. This produces an optimal systolic ejection volume (SEV). The heart VO2 is called the myocardial oxygen consumption or MVO2, (M is for Myocardium). The important point about myocardial oxygen consumption is that the oxygen cost increases exponentially for each increase in heart rate. This is because MVO2 is a squared function of the heart rate.

From all this, we have created an algorithm that allows you to obtain your energy profile from a simple quality GPS-watch measurement. Just to give you an idea, the research required to validate this information was about 45,000 € of equipment per runner, not counting the hundreds of hours of running time spent in the field. Much time and effort have gone into validating the possibility of approaching an energy profile to develop a customized training program. We created the company www.BillaTraining.com to help us finance the costs of teaching graduate students and without having to do fundraising. Interestingly, the average cost of running supplies and entries surpasses one thousand dollars per year, and many runners are hesitant to invest in a training program. The philosophy of BillaTraining.com is to raise your aerobic ceiling so that you are running easier without having to train long distances at the same absolute speed. The marathon will become more enjoyable and pass easier with this reserve of speed you have built.

Most importantly, it gives you the possibility to vary your speed, which allows you to optimize your lactate recycling and creatine phosphate stores. Finally, your running economy will improve with quality strides, a source of elastic energy recovery. A big goal of this BillaTraining.com is to be able to vary your speed during the race and maximize your possibilities of energy regeneration. Adopt the idea of "letting go" in training and competition, as well as in your life!

CHAPTER 16 SUMMARY

CONCEPT: A training program provides a wealth of knowledge and gives the added value of wellness and performance, the two things that makes us the happiest! What we are trying to do at BillaTraining.com is to raise awareness of the concepts of complementarity of the four factors of performance: Power, Cardiac Efficiency, Tolerance to Acidosis and Perception of the physiological load. The Rabit® test allows us to define your physiological characteristics in response to running on your sensations. The energy radar and speed signature are steps past the Rabit® test to individualize and quantify the four pillars of marathon performance.

APPLICATION: The BillaTraining.com method is based on two main principles:

- Respect your racing sensations. It's about giving you the ability to understand your sensations while training and racing accurately. This allows you to avoid over and undertraining, control your running speed in training and competition, maximize your training effectiveness, and set new PR's. Increasing your power reserve is essential to accomplish all of this and to increase the range of your sensations.

- Decrease the quantity of training leading to better recovery and fewer injuries. Most training takes place in 8 to 12-week cycles with a 2-3-week break.

Most athletes in the BillaTraining.com program follow specific sessions of 3-day intervals (Tuesday-Friday, for example), with a long session and at a variable pace (marathon specific). It is important to respect your speed signature, and we always define this at the end of your first training session.

CHAPTER 16

PERSONALIZED TRAINING PROGRAM WITH KEY WORKOUT SESSIONS

IN THIS CHAPTER, WE OFFER you some of the key BillaTraining.com training sessions to develop the four pillars of marathon performance. The sessions are coded according to their difficulty levels. When running to your sensations, training is both fun and effective; it also improves the perception of fatigue and the physiological load of a race. With practice, you will better manage the energy resources in your body consistent with the maintenance of homeostasis, which the balance of the internal environment of our body. One of our goals is to become a good runner, capable of varying speed while maintaining the same comfort "average" zone in the marathon. The energy audit based on the interpretation of the Rabit® test makes it possible to establish your energy profile that characterizes your hybrid engine: Power, Tolerance, Cardiac Reserve, and Perception.

Recall that Power is your alactic anaerobic metabolism or very high-power electric battery. Tolerance to acidosis is the ability to maintain a high level of lactate without "blocking the engine" (which is the second anaerobic lactate battery). The Cardiac Reserve is the supply of oxygen or fuel to feed the thermal engine, and Perception refers to the physiological load (acuteness of the sensations). We possibly would have broken the 2-hour marathon barrier long ago if we agreed to trust the runners in their abilities to vary the speed to their sensations rather than to impose a constant speed.

BILLATRAINING.COM WORKOUTS

We have developed many workouts for runners based on our methods. Most athletes in the BillaTraining.com program follow specific sessions of 3-day intervals (Tuesday, Friday, and Saturday, for example), with a long session at a variable pace (marathon specific). It is important to respect your speed signature, and we always define this at the end of your first training session. Here are just some of our workouts to get you started. For those that want more, perform the Rabit® test and consider signing up for coaching at BillaTraining.com. Level 1 sessions are more suitable for beginner runners (see self-assessment following the Rabit® test) and Level 2 sessions for more experienced runners.

3-minute repeats (level 1 and 2 sessions)

This exercise involves 3-minute repeats at MAS, with 3-minute jog recoveries. Three minutes is about half the time most runners can spend at MAS. This workout is designed to be hard, but not demoralizing. Perform 3-minute repeats as many times as possible; most runners can perform about 5 – 6 in a workout.

30-30s level 1

This exercise involves alternating between 30-second surges at MAS and 30-second jog recoveries. Perform 30-30s for as long as possible. Remember, the point of this exercise is that it allows you to spend nearly 40 percent more time at VO2 max. This is a great exercise for beginners and during the early season. Fifteen to twenty minutes of 30-30s level 1 is usually sufficient.

30-30s level 2

This workout is much more intense than level 1 and is more suitable for experienced runners. After a warmup, start running at 100 percent MAS for 1 minute, which will be about 200 – 400 m. After that fast-paced 1 minute, return to a tempo pace (about 40 percent of MAS), which is about 45 – 60 second/mile slower for 30 seconds. Then you speed back up to 100 percent MAS for 30 seconds and so on. Repeat these 30-30s for as long as you can. The goal is to repeat this process for as long as possible. If you cannot endure 10 minutes of 30-30s V2, you are likely running too fast for the fitness you currently have. Elite runners can run about 3500 – 4000 m during this session.

Perception session

The purpose of a perception session is to learn how to manage one's physical and mental resources. The mind is an excellent sensor of the degree of physical exhaustion with the ability to have the most accurate perception of its physiological load. The ability to anticipate the management of distance and perception are the foundations of the BillaTraining.com method. The stronger these foundations (resource management), the more the sessions on the other three pillars will be useful and beneficial. To drive this point home, our film won a "Green award" at the 2016 Deauville Energy Festival in France. Our film demonstrated the bioenergetic model of speed variation to optimize human metabolism and that it could be transposed to the hybrid car using the theory of biomimicry.

Perception Session level 1

Perception exercises are best used as a test to see how well you perceive your pace without a watch while listening to your body. Consider incorporating these exercises with other workouts. Also, test your self when your legs are fresh and when your legs are 30 minutes into a run. The perfection of the art of variable pace running is mastering these types of exercises.

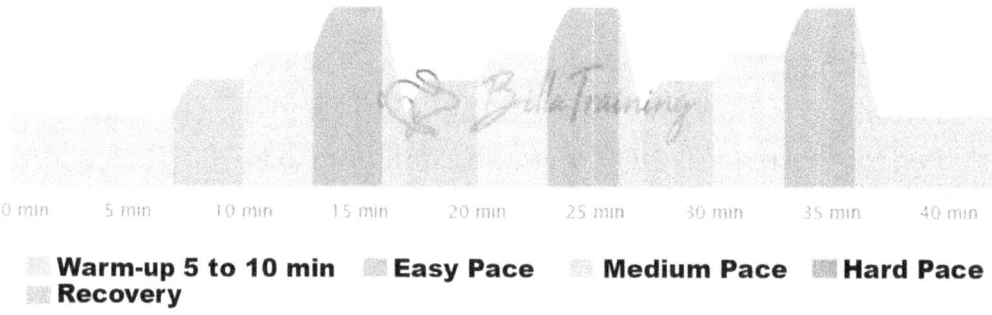

Run four minutes at an easy pace, then two minutes at a medium pace, and then one minute at a hard pace. Finish with three minutes of recuperation. Repeat this exercise three times during a 30-minute run on a flat surface.

Perception Session level 2

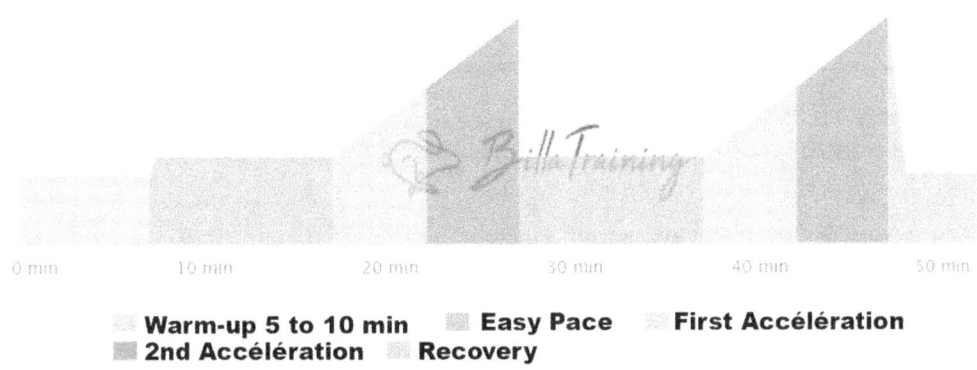

Warm-up 5 to 10 min — Easy Pace — First Accélération
2nd Accélération — Recovery

Run at an easy pace for 10 minutes and then try to accelerate 1 km/hr every minute WITHOUT looking at your watch. Perform these 1-minute accelerations until you are sprinting and then repeat. Download your run and verify on the computer if you succeeded in increasing your speed appropriately using perception alone.

Force-Speed Session (Power)

Training at speeds close to a marathon pace on a constant modality makes you nothing more than a "diesel," i.e., you are unable to change pace with no margin of safety to recover and revive your body once in the red. We have seen previously that power-force (specific to running) plays a crucial role in maintaining momentum without increasing the contact time on the ground. This is important in avoiding putting excess energy into your stride as well as avoiding the excessive use of glycogen. That is why the BillaTraining.com method uses strength and endurance to generate more endurance through specific race sessions. Our goal is to maximize your speed range to create a large power reserve that will allow you to run with a higher margin of safety. Remember that the difference in marathon performance between 2 hours 6 minutes and 36 seconds (Antonio Pinto, European record) and marathoners in the 2 hours and 11 minutes range was correlated with the speed over just 1000-m!

Force-Speed Session level 1

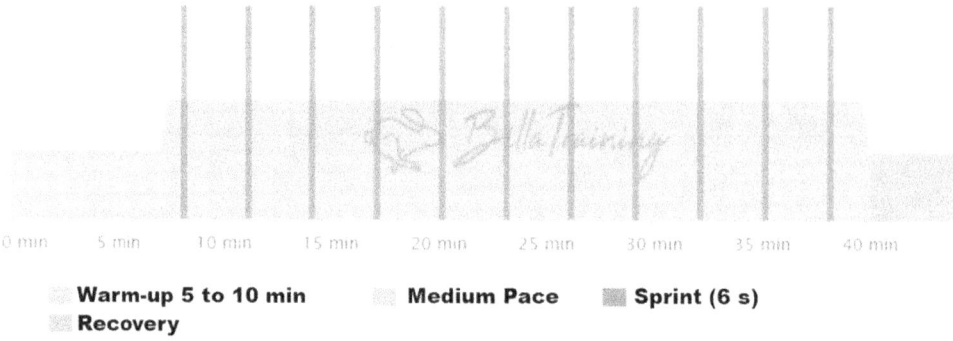

Warm-up 5 to 10 min   Medium Pace   Sprint (6 s)
Recovery

For a workout of 30 minutes, perform accelerations of 4 – 6 seconds every 3 minutes. This training session should be done on a flat surface to work the speed and stride.

Force Speed Session level 2

For a workout of 30 minutes, perform accelerations of 4 – 6 seconds every 3 minutes. This training session should be done on a slight incline (<4 percent). Consider adding 5 percent of body weight via a running vest or camelback to work the speed and stride.

Cardio Sessions

This type of session aims to increase your heart reserve (differential between resting HR and HR max) by developing your heart muscle. The better your cardiac reserve, the more energy you can conserve. Cardiac output (the amount of blood distributed by the heart to the body in a given time) is the product of your heart rate (number of contractions heart rate in one minute) and your volume of systolic ejection (amount of blood expelled at each contraction of the heart). The heart is a muscle. It consumes about 20 percent of the body's oxygen at rest and even more with exercise, as we have seen previously. With each additional heartbeat, the heart consumes a surplus of oxygen, which is oxygen will not go to the muscles. Therefore, it is important to have a "muscular" heart that is efficient and has a large systolic ejection volume. This helps us consume less oxygen per contraction. Another way to think about it is that oxygen becomes more expensive as the exercise level is increased, thus it is about economizing how oxygen is used.

Cardio Session level 1

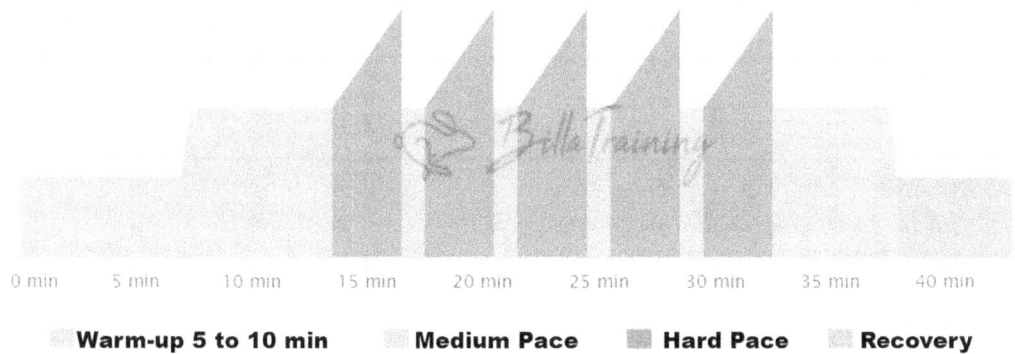

Warm-up 5 to 10 min   Medium Pace   Hard Pace   Recovery

After a warmup, accelerate to your maximal speed over 3 minutes, with one minute of recovery at a medium pace. Repeat this exercise 5 times. You must respect your sensations without trying to reach a certain speed or a goal.

Cardio Session level 2

After a warmup, from a medium pace, accelerate for two minutes to a hard pace, and then deaccelerate two minutes back to a medium pace. Repeat these ten times for a total of 20 minutes. Run on a flat surface.

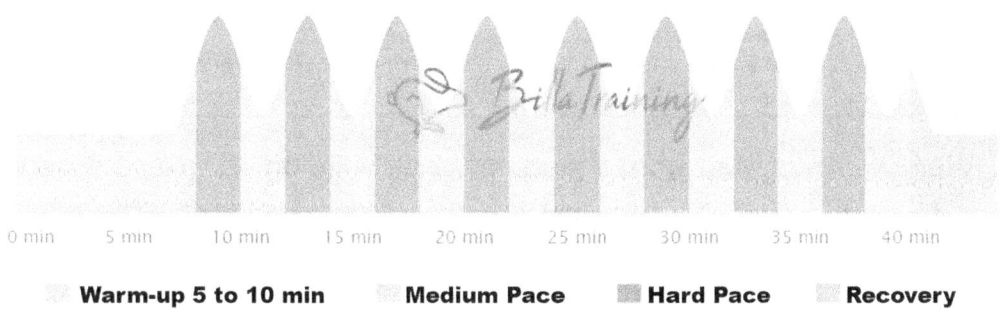

Warm-up 5 to 10 min   Medium Pace   Hard Pace   Recovery

Tolerance to Acidosis Sessions

The goal is to develop your ability to store energy (in the form of lactate) and reuse it to produce a lot of energy at VO2 max and reload the muscles into creatine phosphate.

Tolerance to acidosis session level 1

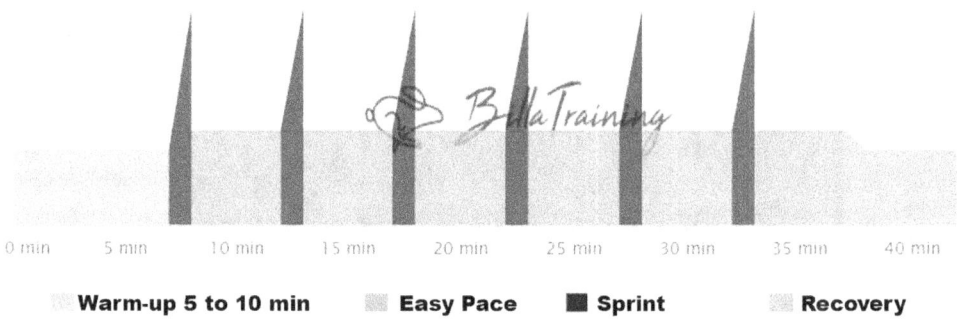

During a 30-minute run, perform 1-minute sprint accelerations to a hard pace, and then recover for four minutes at an easy pace and repeat. Run on a flat surface.

Tolerance to acidosis level 2

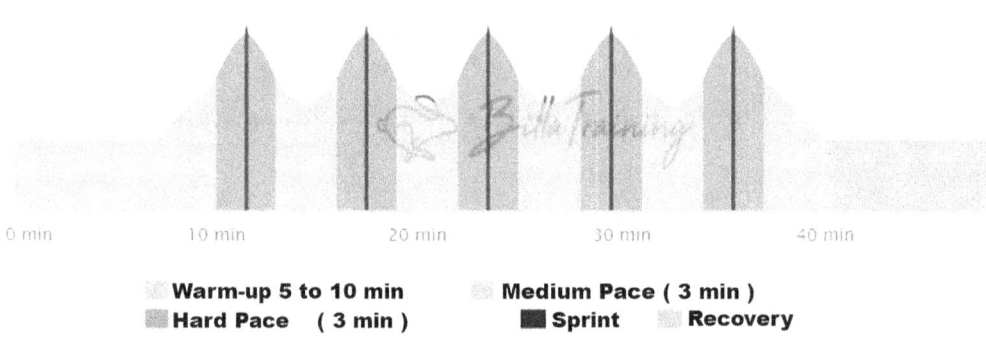

After a warmup, start from a medium pace, building up to a hard pace and hold for 1 minute, and then try to perform a sprint of 10 seconds, and then coming back down to a medium pace. Repeat these five times on a flat surface.

Race technique exercises

These exercises aim to improve propulsive efficiency with a short ground support time, stride, and power optimization while running. For this, we will see different types of exercises aimed at improving posture and coordination.

These exercises are very demanding on the ankles, calves, knees, and thighs. Make sure that you warm up before performing these exercises!

OPTIMIZING FOOT-ANKLE REBOUND EXERCISES

The main goal of these exercises is to optimize the foot-ankle rebound. In French, we call this "d'avoir le pied" or "having the foot." Three aspects are essential to optimize foot placement during running to be more dynamic and to avoid the risk of injury.

1. First, it is important not to directly place your body weight on the heel, also known as a heel strike. The heel is composed of two hard bones (the talus and the calcaneus) and therefore does not allow for shock absorption.

2. The foot must be placed under your center of gravity for optimal foot strike dynamics. When the foot is in front of the center of gravity, there will be a recoil phase that will be detrimental to your performance, in running we call this a heavy stride. Conversely, if the support is located far from the center of gravity, the race economy will be low.

3. Finally, having good ankle range of motion will allow you to be more dynamic and reduce the time of support. To facilitate this, it is recommended to point the tip of the foot slightly towards the sky during the suspension phase.

For the next three exercises, the goal is to go slowly but to make complete gestures.

STATIC FOOT-ANKLE EXERCISE

Learn to differentiate the different parts of the foot by staying first on the heel, then flat, then finally the front of the foot. Then try to quickly move from one part of the foot to the other, starting with the heel to finish on the front of the foot. Naturally, the front of the foot will be more effective.

DYNAMIC FOOT-ANKLE EXERCISE

While moving: In a space of 10 – 15 meters, walk in circles with the following instructions:

1. Stay on the heel. Keep your body straight and take small steps with your legs, looking straight ahead while you are moving your arms.

2. Stay on the front of the foot. Tiptoe as high as possible with the pelvis slightly retroverted. Take small steps with outstretched legs and look forward while using your arms.

3. Unroll the foot as in the static exercise (1) while respecting the objectives of each surface (heel, flat, front). Take small steps with your legs straight. First, perform this exercise by following a line, then zigzagging.

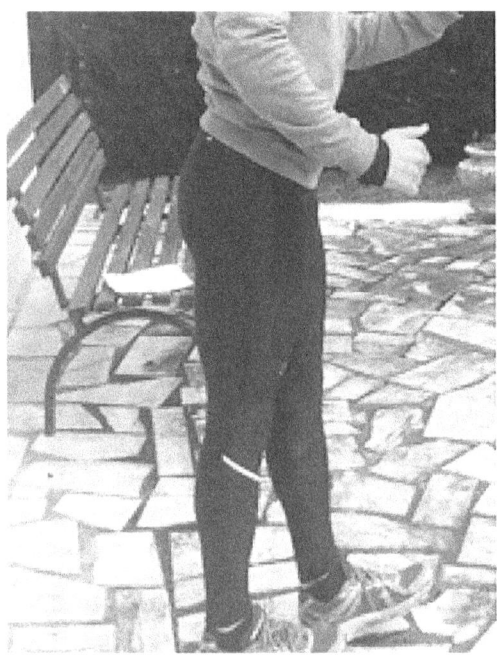
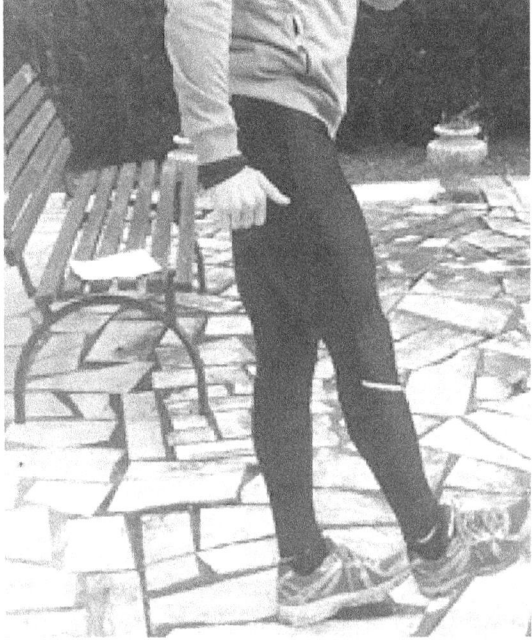

THE KNEES

To get a more effective stride; getting your knees up is essential! The goal is to increase stride and efficiency.

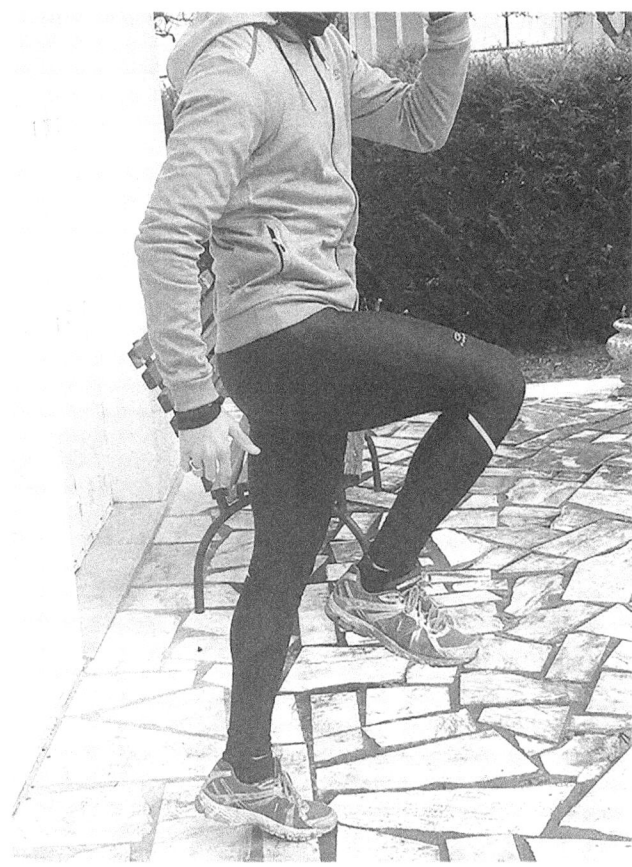

In running, there is a common theme about strides - when fatigue sets in, get the knees up! Practice this exercise before you experience fatigue during the marathon. Exaggerating your stride secondary to fatigue will be expensive energetically. That is why raising your knees in a suitable manner will allow you to increase your stride length. It is important to slightly dampen the knees to avoid significant shocks to the pelvis. For this, when striking the foot on the ground, the knee must be slightly bent and never tense!

Some exercises for the knee:

    Repeat the foot-ankle exercises 2 and 3 of the moving part of the foot, but this time the goal will be to point the knee forward (about 90 degrees). The use of the arms is even more important to balance the body.

Other exercises:

The front slit (pointing the knee forward). This exercise allows you to work different muscle groups such as the femoral quadriceps (in front of the thigh) and the hamstrings (back of the thigh) but also to increase the amplitude of your hip.

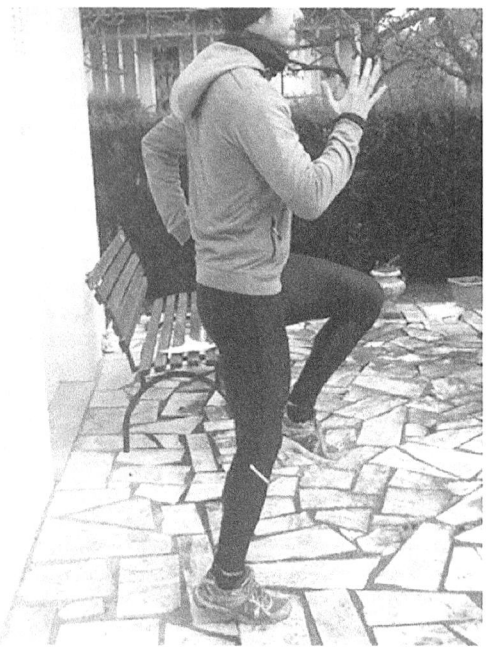
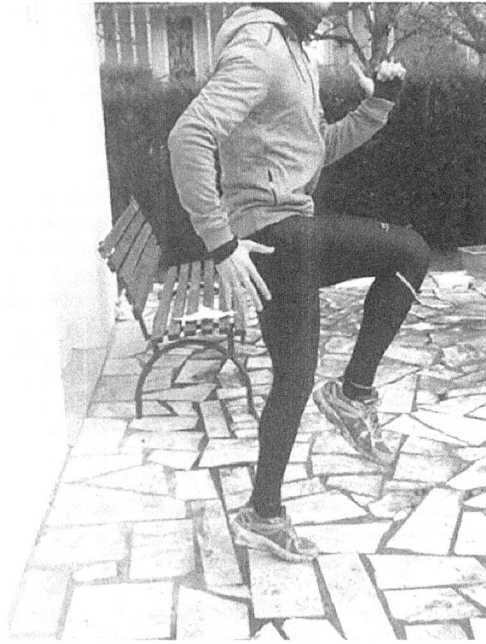
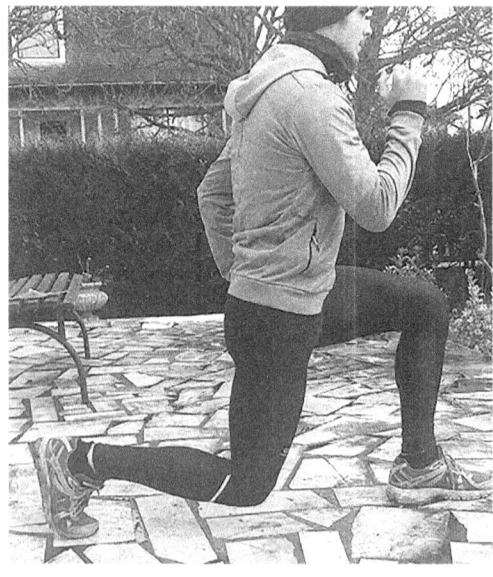

Knee raises are also a good exercise. The goal is to quickly perform knee raises without forward movement. Also keep your abdominal muscles tight during this exercise.

THE PELVIS

The main objective of these pelvic exercises is to optimize the restitution of the power used by the legs. To run efficiently, it is important to keep the whole body upright. For this, the pelvis plays a vital role. Your pelvis must be in a normal position or in a slight retroversion which will facilitate the forward cycle. Being arched (i.e., anteversion) is not suitable for running and is easily identified (the seated runner). Maintaining good alignment helps prevent excessive shocks, which can cause injury.

1st exercise:

> Static: Learn to differentiate the different postures of the pelvis (anteversion/normal/retroversion). A small simple exercise consists in placing one's pelvis successively from retroversion to anteversion. Help yourself by placing your hands on your hips. Once the gesture is acquired, try to observe the most effective posture in running. To do this, look for your knees up in the three postures of the pelvis. Naturally, the retroversion position will be the most effective.

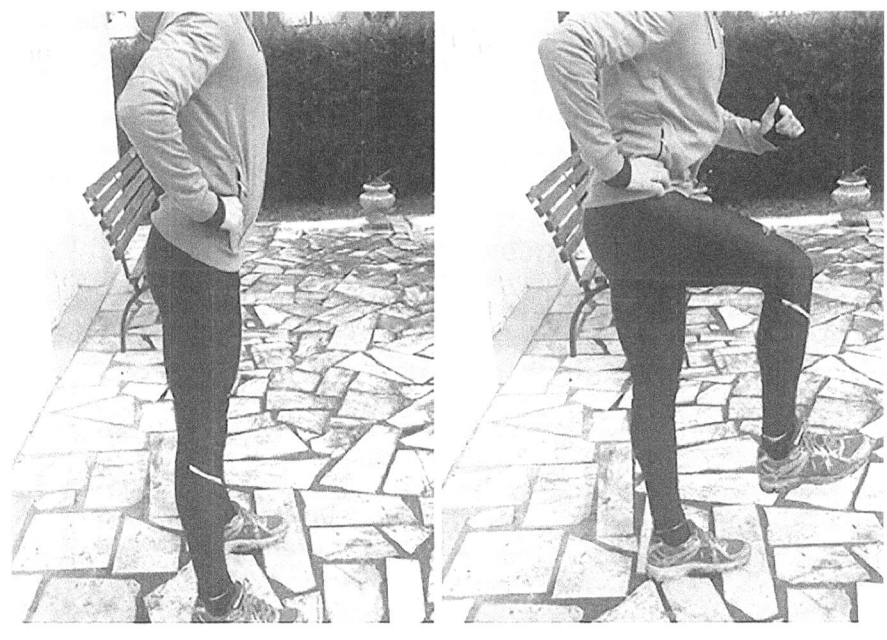

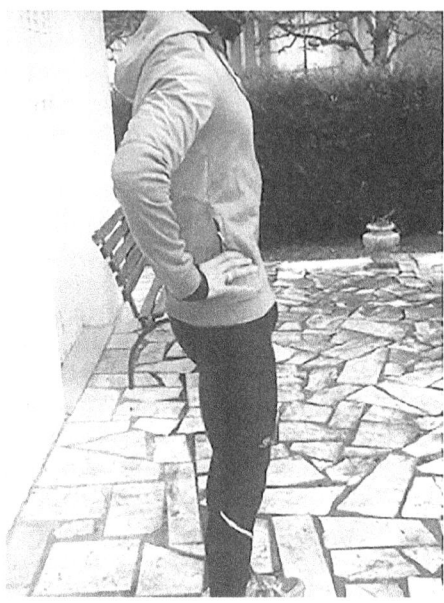 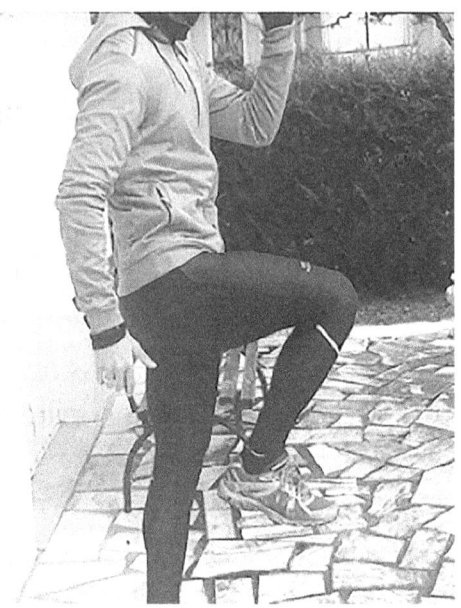

ANTEVERSION AND RETROVERSION OF THE PELVIS

2nd exercise: Stand on the front of the foot. While standing one knee, focus on the pelvis and being tall (12 seconds on each leg).

WALKING EXERCISES.

While walking up steps, place one leg on the upper step, and then push on that leg to go as high as possible by pointing the knee forward dynamic using the arms (Ten repetitions of each leg).

Nasal Breathing

An often-overlooked exercise is nasal breathing. The body naturally does better with nasal breathing. Our noses are specifically designed part of our respiratory system and has many health benefits.

Nasal breathing facts:

- Ensures better blood flow and lung volumes
- Warms and filters air
- Better maintenance of body temperature

- 10 – 20% Improved oxygen uptake
- Prevents sleep apnea
- Decreases infections
- 75% population has a deviated septum
- May help exercise induced asthma.
- Tolerance to acidosis improves
- Tolerance to CO_2 buildup improves
- Help asthma
- Temperature is better regulated when you learn to breath nasally

There are many breathing methods and it is important to become good at one. Breathing is a mental practice, and that is why it is often difficult for people to master these techniques. A research study showed that if your nasal passages are chronically blocked, the risk of sleep apnea, sinus infections, and overall health diminishes. What is worse if you only breath through your mouth. Think of the nasal passages as a muscle. If you do not use your nasal passages, they will shrink. It takes time to become used to nasal breathing, but one you do it, you will feel more at ease. If you are a recreational runner, consider nasal breathing all the time. If you feel like you are not getting enough air, then switch and try it again. If you are an elite runner, you will need to use nose and mouth breathing at different times.

A couple of exercises to consider is to practice breathing thirty times and then hold your breath. This builds up your tolerance to carbon dioxide.

- During a threshold run, practice nasal breathing for some minutes at a time. You will find that you will become more comfortable with nasal breathing quickly.
- Practice 6-second drills. Inhale for 6 seconds, and exhale for 6 seconds.
- A new book, *Breath*, written by James Nestor is a good read.
- As breathing guru Wim Hoff says, just breath!!

HOW TO PERFORM A PROPER SQUAT

The squat is essential to our wellbeing and is a natural fundamental human movement. A proper squat movement can greatly improve your power reserve and keep your hips, back, and knees healthy as we age. The squat position is nature's intended sitting position, and there is nothing artificial about this movement. It is a hip flexion and extension exercise.

The feet should be about shoulder's width, head up, the back should be normally arched, and abdominals are tight. Sending your buttocks and back down, be sure the knees track over the line of the feet, not allowing the knees to roll inside. Keep pressure on the heels and maintain good posture. A proper squat involves you "pulling" yourself down with your hip flexors, not letting gravity dropping you to the ground. Stop when your hips are slightly below the knees. Then return up on the exact path which you came down. Focus on using every bit of musculature possible and finally stand as tall as possible. Try performing air squats. Many gyms focus on teaching the squat technique as it is a fundamental movement to just about every exercise. Perform at least ten air squats per day with perfect form. Have someone else observe your movements or record them on your phone. Some causes of poor squat technique are weak gluteal and hamstring muscles, poor muscular engagement, and weak control.

CHAPTER 15 SUMMARY

CONCEPT: Training according to your sensations is both fun and effective, improves the perception fatigue and the physiological load of a race. With practice you will better manage the energy resources in your body consistent with the maintenance of homeostasis which the balance of the internal environment of our body. The Rabit® test makes it possible to establish your energy profile that characterizes your four pillars of marathon running: Power, Tolerance, Cardiac Reserve, and Perception. Power is your alactic anaerobic metabolism or very high-power electric battery. Tolerance to acidosis or the ability to maintain a high level of lactate without "blocking the engine." The Cardiac Reserve is the supply of oxygen and fuel. Perception relates to the physiological load (acuteness of the sensations).

APPLICATION: In this book, we offer you some key BillaTraining.com training sessions to develop the four pillars of marathon performance. The sessions are coded according to their difficulty levels. Level 1 sessions are more suitable for beginner runners (see self-assessment following the Rabit® test) and Level 2 sessions for more experienced runners. The energy audit based on the interpretation of the Rabit® test makes it possible to establish your energy profile that characterizes your hybrid engine: Power, Tolerance, Cardiac Reserve, and Perception.

CHAPTER 17

DEVELOPING YOUR SPEED SIGNATURE FOR MARATHON DAY

BEFORE WE DIVE INTO DEVELOPING your speed signature, it is worth reviewing this book's fundamental points. Since 1990, we have worked hard developing these "old school" concepts to bring back the art of variable pace running. We have summarized more than twenty-five years of the beginnings of a small personal scientific revolution! With a better understanding of physiological adaptations to exercise, it becomes apparent that we are meant to run using frequency and variation. We need to be allowed to run free. To move forward, we always remind our runners and research colleagues to overcome these ideas of constant pace training that have slowed us down. By identifying our speeds, we can use time and intensity to characterize the energy demands that can serve as benchmarks for constructing a personalized training program. As an internationally acclaimed professor in exercise physiology, Dr. Billat has freed herself from the traditional research of constant speed to move towards acceleration models (positive and negative). Finally, running a marathon using our sensations is the goal.

Here is a short timeline of Dr. Billat's journey:

- 1985-88: The lactate threshold exists only in an incremental VAMEVAL type protocol. It is preferable to look for the maximum steady-state velocity of lactate over time: training at this speed of stable state of lactate makes it possible to run for thirty minutes and increases the MCT enzyme lactate transporters.

- 1990-1995: The MAS and VO2 max are insufficient to characterize the energy profile of a runner. It is necessary to determine the runner's time limit at MAS and develop his/her interval training as a percentage of the time limit at MAS. With the addition of the possibility to use the sessions of short intervals like the 15-15s, which makes it possible to solicit phosphocreatine by stimulating oxidative phosphorylation and shuttle creatine kinase. Creatine phosphate is used for the contraction of myofibrils. We already knew that creatine phosphate could serve as a substrate in short intervals with active recovery intervals at fifty percent HR max. It should be remembered that the myocardium has an LDH-H (H) enzyme that recycles lactate into pyruvic acid and is then oxidized for energy.

- 2000: Using a portable gas exchange gas analyzer, Dr. Billat's laboratory determined the velocity requiring the maximum energy at VO2 max by running measuring the time limits between 90 – 140 percent MAS. This allowed us to take into account only the time spent at VO2 max and therefore, the energy supplied by VO2 max and the distance traveled at VO2 max. This critical speed at VO2 max corresponded to the minimum speed associated with VO2 max in a VAMEVAL type protocol but with large variations between the runners (between 95 – 110% of MAS). This meant that the maximum energy produced at VO2 max was at 95 – 105% MAS, depending on the runner. Also, the components of VO2 max (cardiac output and oxygen arterio-venous difference) are not maximized according to the velocities requiring VO2 max.

- 2006: An interesting experiment is to run 10-km using a variable pace strategy and then measure your average speed. Then run that same distance, but at a constant pace with the same average speed, and you will find that in most cases, you will only be able to hold that pace for about 7000-m. Dr. Billat showed this in a 2006 research paper. A constant speed 10-km run resulted in higher oxygen consumption, higher average heart rate, higher HR max, and increased metabolic cost than the free-run group. Allowing the runner to vary his speed frees the metabolism to fluctuate between anaerobic and aerobic glycolysis, optimizing the recycling of lactate and creatine phosphate synthesis. Many runners choose a cadence that gives comfort, but not necessarily the best race economy.

- 2010: Dr. Billat began to move away from the constant speed running model (expressed as a percentage of MAS, for example). Indeed, newer technologies such as high-performance GPS have allowed us to verify that the best racing performances are not achieved at a constant speed. In addition, depending on distances and training times, the actual speed varies greatly.

- 2015: To determine the maximum energy at VO2 max and its associated speed, we highlighted that the energy at VO2 max provided about 30 percent of the energy during a 100-m race for elite sprinters; and VO2 max provided about 50 percent of the energy over a 3000-m race and only 10 percent for the marathon. However, our data only applied to mid-level marathoners (3.5 hours).

- 2018: Acceleration-based training improved performance, cardiac function, muscle mechanics, optimized metabolic, and cellular adaptions in an 8-week program. Acceleration-based training also decreases training time and injuries as well as prevents sarcopenia in older mice. Finally, acceleration-based training increases the power reserve, which is essential for running your marathon without cracking and with all the pleasure of running it below your average speed for over half of the race. Running a marathon using speed variations is the key to finishing the event and enjoying the experience.

Certainly, we can now offer a new method of training for the marathon. We can run faster by using our ability to feel and control the pace without thinking. Our race strategies will not help us when we are trying to get from point A to B in an actual marathon in the best time possible. We are not machines with predictive control loops in anticipatory action. Recall that force is the ability to accelerate a mass, Newton's definition of unity. It will no longer be necessary to train many miles to achieve fractional improvements. We want to free the runner from the stress of not being able to run the eighth 200-m in a specific time.

In conclusion, it took a quarter of a century to change the ideas of constant pace running. We hope that this book will save you time running and avoid the inutile physiological debates that abound on the internet. The marathon is a powerful generator of sensory experiences that we have blurred with numbers and dogmatic scientific approaches. We have shown that the records (at all levels of performance) can be beaten using variable speed if we examine the running speeds via a GPS-watch. The best running performance is not achieved at a constant speed but variable speeds. Indeed, every mile or kilometer time point hides large variations that are specific to each runner. Be able to understand its hidden meaning by analyzing the successive physiological states of these variations of speed. The goal of the race is to be able to finish without early fatigue without putting oneself in danger, beyond the limits of our physiological constants (glycemia, temperature, dehydration, acidosis., etc.).

FUNDAMENTAL POINT N ° 1: VARIABLE SPEED

On this point, it is clear: the successful races are carried out with a fast start, then a decrease in speed followed by variations of speed. Near the end of the marathon, the runner will have the ability to reaccelerate to the same level of their starting speed. Numerous statistics and scientific research support these claims. To schematize this point, it evokes that we must run-in a U-shaped pattern. In other words, having a fast start above the average target speed, then most of the race slightly below the average target speed, and a new acceleration at the end of the race above the average target speed. The strategy is to start quickly and "do not resist the euphoria of the start" and let go and find your pace of comfort and reaccelerate near the end.

FUNDAMENTAL POINT N ° 2: INCREASE YOUR SPEED RESERVE

The key to success is through an increase of muscular strength! This is what we have been saying for years now. To run a fast marathon, one must also be capable of running a fast 10-km. It goes even further by saying that we must develop power over 10 and 30 seconds. It is this power that, in addition to allowing you to withstand fatigue, will allow you to withstand a quick start. To develop this power, Dr. Billat proposes three simple to follow types of accelerations: soft, medium, and strong.

FUNDAMENTAL POINT N° 3: MINIMALIST AND QUALITATIVE TRAINING

Dr. Billat has studied for more than 30 years the science of running. She points out the benefits of variable-paced training, and the disadvantages of constant-paced training: monotony, high volume, the imposition of one-pace. To make training as efficient as possible and avoid injuries (for the master's runner in particular), integrate accelerations of 10 seconds starting from a medium speed zone by repeating them; 10 times every 3 minutes, for example.

FUNDAMENTAL POINT N° 4: LISTENING TO YOUR SENSATIONS

Putting sensations back at the center of the training process is one of the pillars of BillaTraining.com. It's about giving you back the ability to control your racing speed in training and competition. This comes first and foremost by a test called the RABIT, an acronym for *Running Advisor BillaTraining*, which is based on sensations and accelerations interspersed with minutes of recovery. We must take back our primacy to sensations and variable speeds with no more imposed speeds and constant-speed-high-mileage traditional training plans.

FUNDAMENTAL POINT N° 5: VARIABLE SPEED TRAINING

The last key of the BillaTraining.com secret lies in variable speeds in competition and training. Each session must incorporate variations in speed within the body of the session.

- Example of perception session: 3 x (4 min at endurance / 2 min pace at marathon pace/1 min at MAS)

- Example of strength/speed session: 4 – 6 seconds of acceleration every 3 minutes within 30 minutes at marathon pace

- Example of cardio efficiency session: 5 x (3 min in acceleration up to MAS/1 min at marathon pace)

- Example of tolerance session to acidosis: 6 x (4 min in endurance/1 min of sprint in acceleration)

DEVELOPING YOUR SPEED SIGNATURE

Your speed signature is the culmination of your physiology, running economy, psychology, metabolism, and performance. Think of your speed signature as to what you know how to do innately during the marathon. The speed signature is a combination of strategies and feedbacks during the race based on physiological and mental feelings. The result of the Rabit® test allows you to devise a speed variation strategy to achieve the best possible time given your current energy profile. We want a performance to be considered in these two dimensions: a realistic time for the marathon and the way to achieve it. Remember that a straight line is the shortest path from one point to another, provided that the two points are in front of each other (Pierre Dac).

What this comes down to is that the most effective and least arduous way to run will be to take advantage of your fresh muscles by starting quickly. Then gradually reduce your speed to cover the most kilometers below your final average speed as defined according to your performance objectives. Your marathon race strategy starts at the highest speed of your so-called "medium" comfort zone. You will then vary your speeds (make waves) by staying in this zone between the highest and the lowest speeds. The comfort speed zone "medium" is the speed to use on the marathon. Finally, you will slightly increase your pace over the last two kilometers (remember the U-shaped racing strategies). By using this strategy, you will not only run faster than you do while running at a constant speed, but you will also recover three times faster (3 weeks instead of 9 weeks). Indeed, the marathon "leaves deep muscular tracks" when it is run steadily up to a limit that will often hit the famous 30th-km where the speed and energy run out.

THE TEN GOLDEN RULES OF THE WWW.BILLATRAINING.COM METHOD

In conclusion, here are the ten golden rules before you start to live by the BillaTraining.com method. It is necessary to follow the following rules for at least 12 weeks for the best results.

1. Perform a Strength, Cardio, Acidosis, or Perception session 2 or 3 times a week separated by 48-hours. For example, perform a Force session on Tuesday, a Perception session on Friday.

2. Long run on Sunday. This training can be free (distance, time, etc.) or a repetition of your personal speed signature. During the 1 – 3-hour free run/walk, try to keep your sensations in mind and vary your speed from easy to a sprint during each of these sessions.

3. On Wednesday, run a tolerance-to-acidosis session. Then on Saturday, run a perception session. On Sunday, a long run using your speed signature (which we also propose to calculate in the 3-month program at www.BillaTraining.com).

4. If you do not want to do a workout for various reasons (busy workday, fatigue, etc.), do not do it and move to the next day.

5. The specific sessions should last about 30 minutes. Since they are based on perception, you will be sure to focus on yourself, and it is best to run alone.

6. Do not watch your GPS-watch while running, stay focused on your sensations, and analyze your curve after the training that corresponds to your difficulty level.

7. Finding the time to watch a movie, have a family meal, play an online video game, read a good book, are all integral parts of the training. By having time to do these things, you will be more than happy to train and compete. How many runners find themselves on the starting line early on a Sunday morning wondering, "what are they doing here?"

8. The variety of sessions is what promotes progress and prevents overtraining.

9. Experiment with your sessions and share them with us because we do not hold the absolute truth! Just as the present is only worth the intensity, we must live in the moment. The race makes us more palpable to the moment.

10. Dare to be different, and above all, enjoy yourself!

BIBLIOGRAPHY

Ahmaidi S, Adam, C Préfaut C. Validité des épreuves triangulaires de course navette de 20-m et de course sur piste pour l'estimation de la consommation maximale d'oxygène du sportif. Science et Sports 5, 71-76, 1990.

Ahmaidi S, Collomp K, Préfaut C. The effect of shuttle test protocol and the resulting lactacidemia on maximal velocity and maximal oxygen uptake during the shuttle exercise test. Eur J Appl Physiol 65, 475-479, 1992a.

Ahmaidi S, Collomp K, Caillaud C, Préfaut C. Maximal and functional aerobic capacity as assessed by two graduated field methods in comparison to laboratory exercise testing in moderately trained subjects. Int J Sports Med 13, 243-248, 1992b.

Aliev M, Guzun R, Karu-Varikmaa M, Kaambre T, Wallimann T, Saks V. Molecular system bioenergics of the heart: experimental studies of metabolic compartmentation and energy fluxes versus computer modeling. Int J Mol Sci 12, 9296-9331, 2011.

Antonini MT, Billat V, Blanc P, Chassain AP, Dalmay F, Menier R, Virot P. Comparaison de la lactatémie en régime transitoire et en régime stationnaire d'exercice musculaire. Science et Sport 2, 41-44, 1987.

Astrand PO, Ryhming I., A nomogram for calculation of aerobic capacity (physical fitness) from pulse rate during sub-maximal work. J Appl Physiol 7, 218-221, 1954.

Astrand PO, Saltin B. Oxygen uptake during the first minutes of heavy muscular exercise. J Appl Physiol 16, 971-976, 1961.

Aunola S, Rusko H. Reproducibility of aerobic and anaerobic thresholds in 20-50-year-old men. Eur J Appl Physiol Occup Physiol 53, 260-266, 1984.

Baldwin KM, Cooke DA, Cheadle WG. Time course adaptations in cardiac and skeletal muscle to different running programs. J Appl Physiol Respir Environ Exerc Physiol 42, 267-272, 1977.

Baquet G, Berthoin S, Gerbeaux M, Van Praagh E. Assessment of maximal aerobic speed with an incremental running field test in children. Biol Sport 16, 23-30, 1999.

Barauna VG, Magalhaes FC, Krieger JE, Oliveira EM. AT1 receptor participates in the cardiac hypertrophy induced by resistance training in rats. Am J Physiol Regul Integr Comp Physiol 295, R381-387, 2008.

Baron B, Moullan F, Deruelle F, Noakes TD. The role of emotions on pacing strategies and performance in middle and long duration sport events. Br J Sports Med 45, 511517, 2011.

Bernard C. Leçons sur les propriétés physiologiques et les altérations pathologiques des liquides de l'organisme, Baillères JB & Fils, Paris, Tome I, 524 pages, 1859.

Berthoin S, Gerbeaux M, Guerrin F, Lensel-Corbeil G, Vandendorpe F. Estimation de la Vitesse Maximale Aérobie. Science et Sports, 85-91, 1992.

Berthoin S, Gerbeaux M, Guerrin F, Lensel-Corbeil G, Turpin E, Vandendorpe F. Comparison of two field tests to estimate maximum aerobic speed. J Sports Sci 12, 355362, 1994.

Berthoin S, Mantéca F, Gerbeaux M, Lensel-Corbeil G. Effect of a 12-week training program on Maximal Aerobic Speed (MAS) and running time to exhaustion at 100 % of MAS for students aged 14 to 17 years. J Sports Med Phys Fitness 35, 251-256, 1995.

Berthoin S, Baquet G, Manteca F, Lensel-Corbeil G, Gerbeaux M. Maximal aerobic speed and running time to exhaustion for children 6 to 17 years old. Ped Exerc Sci 8, 234-244, 1996a.

Berthoin S, Pelayo P, Lensel-Corbeil G, Robin H, Gerbeaux M. Comparison of maximal aerobic speed as assessed with laboratory and field measurements in moderately trained subjects. Int J Sports Med 17, 525-529, 1996b.

Berthoin S, Baquet G, Rabita J, Blondel N, Lensel-Corbeil G, Gerbeaux M. Validity of the Université de Montréal Track Test to assess the velocity associated with peak oxygen uptake for adolescents. J Sports Med Phys Fitness 39,107-112, 1999.

Berthon P, Fellmann N, Bedu M, Beaune B, Dabonneville M, Coudert J, Chamoux A. A 5-min running field test as a measurement of maximal aerobic velocity. Eur J Appl Physiol Occup Physiol 75, 233-238, 1997.

Bigard AX, Sanchez H, Koulmann N. Modulations du génome exprimé dans le muscle squelettique avec l'entraînement physique. Science & Sports 22, 267–279, 2007.

Billat V. Physiologie et méthodologie de l'entraînement. De Boeck Supérieur, Bruxelles, Belgique, 4e édition, 296 pages, 2017.

Billat V. Révolution Marathon. De Boeck Supérieur, Bruxelles, Belgique, 4e édition, 208 pages, 2018.

Billat LV. Use of blood lactate measurements for prediction of exercise performance and for control of training. Recommendations for long-distance running. Sports Med 22, 157-175, 1996.

Billat LV, Koralsztein JP. Significance of the velocity at VO2max and time to exhaustion at this velocity. Sports Med 22, 90-108, 1996.

Billat V, Renoux JC, Pinoteau J, Petit B, Koralsztein JP. Validation d'une épreuve de temps limite à VMA (vitesse maximale aérobie) et à VO2max. Science et Sports 9, 135143, 1994a.

Billat V, Bernard O, Pinoteau J, Petit B, Koralsztein JP. Time to exhaustion at VO2max and lactate steady state velocity in sub elite long-distance runners. Arch Int Physiol Biochim Biophys 102, 215-219, 1994b.

Billat V, Dalmay F, Antonini MT, Chassain AP. A method for determining the maximal steady state of blood lactate concentration from two levels of submaximal exercise. Eur J Appl Physiol Occup Physiol 69, 196-202, 1994c.

Billat V, Renoux JC, Pinoteau J, Petit B, Koralsztein JP. Reproducibility of running time to exhaustion at VO2max in subelite runners. Med Sci Sports Exerc 26, 254-257, 1994d.

Billat VL, Hill DW, Pinoteau J, Petit B, Koralsztein JP. Effect of protocol on determination of velocity at VO2max and on its time to exhaustion. Arch Physiol Biochem 104, 313-21, 1996a.

Billat V, Petit B, Koralsztein JP. Calibration de la durée des répétitions d'une séance d'interval training à la vitesse associée à VO2max en référence au temps limite continu: effet sur les réponses physiologiques et la distance parcourue. Science et Motricité 28, 13-20, 1996b.

Billat VL, Flechet B, Petit B, Muriaux G, Koralsztein JP. Interval training at VO2max: effects on aerobic performance and overtraining markers. Med Sci Sports Exerc 31, 156-163, Eur J Appl Physiol Occup Physiol 80, 159-61, 1999a.

Billat VL, Blondel N, Berthoin S. Determination of the velocity associated with the longest time to exhaustion at maximal oxygen uptake. Eur J Appl Physiol Occup Physiol 80, 159-161, 1999b.

Billat V, Blondel N, Berthoin S. The velocity associated with VO2max for all supa critical run is the velocity which elicits the longest time to exhaustion at VO2max. Eur J Appl Physiol 80, 159-161, 2000.

Billat V, Berthoin S, Blondel N, Gerbeaux M. La vitesse à VO2max, signification et applications en course à pied. STAPS 54, 45-61, 2001a.

Billat VL, Demarle A, Slawinski J, Paiva M, Koralsztein JP. Physical and training characteristics of top-class marathon runners. Med Sci Sports Exerc 33, 2089-2097, 2001b.

Billat VL, Wesfreid E, Kapfer C, Koralsztein JP, Meyer Y. Nonlinear dynamics of heart rate and oxygen uptake in exhaustive 10,000 m runs: influence of constant vs. freely paced. J Physiol Sci. 56, 103–111, 2006.

Billat V, Hamard L, Koralsztein JP, Morton RH. Differential modeling of anaerobic and aerobic metabolism in the 800m and 1500m run. J Appl Physiol 107, 478-87, 2009.

Billat VL, Petot H, Landrain M, Meilland R, Koralsztein JP, Mille-Hamard L. Cardiac output and performance during a marathon race in middle-aged recreational runners. Scientific World Journal. 2012.

Billat V, Petot H, Karp JR, Sarre G, Morton RH, Mille-Hamard L. The sustainability of VO2max: effect of decreasing the workload. Eur J Appl Physiol 113, 85-394, 2013.

Billat V, Dhonneur G, Mille-Hamard L, Le Moyec L, Momken I, Launay T, Koralsztein JP, Besse S. Case Studies in Physiology: Maximal oxygen consumption and performance in a centenarian cyclist. J Appl Physiol 122, 430-434, 2017.

Billat V, Brunel N J-B, Carbillet T, Labbé S, Samson A. Humans are able to self-paced constant running accelerations until exhaustion. Physica A 506, 290-304, 2018.

Blondel N, Berthoin S, Billat V, Lensel G. Relationship between run times to exhaustion at 90, 100, 120, and 140% of vVO2max and velocity expressed relatively to critical velocity and maximal velocity. Int J Sports Med 22, 27-33, 2001.

Borg G. Perceived exertion as an indicator of somatic stress. Scand J Rehabil Med 2, 92-98, 1970. Borg GA. Psychophysical bases of perceived exertion. Med Sci Sports Exerc 14, 377381, 1982.

Brandou F, Savy-Pacaux AM, Marie J, Bauloz M, Maret-Fleuret I, Borrocoso S, Mercier J, Brun JF. Impact of high- and low-intensity targeted exercise training on the type of substrate utilization in obese boys submitted to a hypocaloric diet. Diabetes Meta 31, 327-335, 2005.

Brass EP, Scarrow AM, Ruff LJ, Masterson KA, Van Lunteren E. Carnitine delays rat skeletal muscle fatigue in vitro. J Appl Physiol 75, 1595-1600, 1993.

Brooks GA. Anaerobic threshold: review of the concept and directions for future research. Med Sci Sports Exerc 17, 22-34, 1985.

Brooks GA. The lactate shuttle during exercise and recovery. Med Sci Sports Exerc 18, 360-368, 1986.

Brooks G.A., Mercier J. Balance of carbohydrate and lipid utilization during exercise: the « crossover » concept. J. Appl. Physiol 76, 2253-2261, 1994.

Cazorla G. Tests de terrain pour évaluer la capacité aérobie et la vitesse maximale aérobie. In G. Cazorla et G. Robert (Coord.), L'évaluation en activité physique et en sport, 151-174, Cestas, AREAPS, 1990.

Chamoux A, Berthon P, Laubignat, JF. Determination of maximum aerobic velocity by a five-minute test with reference to running world records. A theoretical approach. Arch Int Physiol 104, 207-211, 1996.

Chassain A.P. Méthodes d'appréciation objective de la tolérance de l'organisme à l'effort : application à la mesure des puissances critiques de la fréquence cardiaque et de la lactatémie. Science et Sport 1, 41-48, 1986.

Conconi F, Ferrari M, Ziglio PG, Droghetti P, Codeca L. Determination of the anaerobic threshold by a noninvasive field test in runners. J Appl Physiol Respir Environ Exerc Physiol 52, 869-873, 1982.

Conley DL, Krahenbuhl GS. Running economy and distance running performance of highly trained athletes. Med Sci Sports Exerc 12, 357-360, 1980.

Cooper KH. Aerobics. Bantam Books, New York, USA, 182 pages, 1968. Damasio A, Carvalho GB. The nature of feelings: evolutionary and neurobiological origins. Nat Rev Neurosci 14, 43-52, 2013.

Daniels J, Scardina N, Hayes J, Foley P. Elite and subelite female middle- and long-distance runners. Lander DM (Ed), Sport and elite performers. Human Kinetics, Champaign Il, USA, 57-72 pages, 1984.

Daniels J. A physiologist's view of running economy. Medicine and Science in Sports and Exercise, 17, 332-338, 1985.

Daniels J. Daniels' Formula. Human Kinetics Publisher. Champaign IL, USA, 320 pages, 2014.

Daries HN, Noakes TD, Dennis SC. Effect of fluid intake volume on 2-h running performances in a 25 degrees C environment. Med Sci Sports Exerc 32, 1783-1789, 2000.

Davis HA, Bassett J, Hughes P, Gass GC. Anaerobic threshold and lactate turn point. Eur J Appl Physiol Occup Physiol 50, 383-392, 1983.

Denis C, Dormois D, Castells J, Bonnefoy R, Padilla S, Geyssant A, Lacour JR. Comparison of incremental and steady state tests of endurance training. Eur J Appl Physiol Occup Physiol 57, 474-81, 1988.

di Prampero PE, Atchou G, Brückner JC, Moia C. The energetics of endurance running. The energetics of endurance running. Eur J Appl Physiol Occup Physiol 55, 259266, 1986.

di Prampero PE, Capelli C, Pagliaro P, Antonutto G, Girardis M, Zamparo P, Soule

R G. Energetics of best performances in middle-distance running. J Appl Physiol 74, 23182324, 1993.

Donovan CM, Brooks GA. Endurance training affects lactate clearance, not lactate production. Am J Physiol 244, E83-92, 1983.

Dzeja PP, Terzic A. Phospho-transfer networks and cellular energetics. J Exp Biol 206, 2039-2047, 2003.

Dzeja PP, Zeleznikar RJ, Goldberg ND. Suppression of creatine kinase-catalyzed phosphotransfer results in increased phosphoryl transfer by adenylate kinase in intact skeletal muscle. J Biol Chem 271, 12847-12851, 1996.

Dzeja PP, Terzic A, Wieringa B. Phospho-transfer dynamics in skeletal muscle from creatine kinase gene-deleted mice. Mol Cell Biochem 256-257 (1-2), 13-27, 2004.

Dzeja PP, Hoyer K, Tian R, Zhang S, Nemutlu E, Spindler M, Ingwall JS. Rearrangement of energetic and substrate utilization networks compensate for chronic myocardial creatine kinase deficiency. J Physiol 589 (Pt 21)193-211, 2011.

Edwards RH. Human muscle function and fatigue. Ciba Found Symp 82, 1-18, 1981. Erdmann WS, Lipinska P. Kinematics of marathon running tactics. Hum Mov Sci 32, 1379-1392, 2013.

Ernst MO, Bülthoff HH. Merging the senses into a robust percept. Trends Cogn Sci 8, 162-169, 2004.

Essen B. Studies on the regulation of metabolism in human skeletal muscle using intermittent exercise as an experimental model. Acta Physiol. Scand. (suppl) 454, 7-32, 1978.

Eston RG, Lamb KL, Parfitt G, King N. The validity of predicting maximal oxygen uptake from a perceptually regulated graded exercise test. Eur J Appl Physiol 94, 221-227, 2005.

Eston R. Use of ratings of perceived exertion in sports. Int J Sports Physiol Perform 7, 175-182, 2012.

Ettema JH. Limits of human performance and energy-production. Int J Angew Physiol Einschl Arbeit Physiol 22, 45-54, 1966.

Faina M, Billat V, Squadrone R, De Angelis M, Koralsztein JP, Dal Monte A.

Anaerobic contribution to the time to exhaustion at the minimal exercise intensity at which maximal oxygen uptake occurs in elite cyclists, kayakists and swimmers. Eur J Appl Physiol Occup Physiol 76, 13-20, 1997.

Farrell PA, Wilmore JH, Coyle EF, Billing JE, Costill DL. Plasma lactate accumulation and distance running performance. Med Sci Sports 11, 338-344, 1979.

Favier RJ, Constable SH, Chen M, Holloszy JO. Endurance exercise training reduces lactate production. J Appl Physiol 61, 885-889, 1986.

Figueiredo PA, Powers SK, Ferreira RM, Appell HJ, Duarte JA. Aging impairs skeletal muscle mitochondrial bioenergetic function. J Gerontol A Biol Sci Med Sci 64, 21-33, 2009a.

Figueiredo PA, Powers SK, Ferreira RM, Amado F, Appell HJ, Duarte JA. Impact of lifelong sedentary behavior on mitochondrial function of mice skeletal muscle. J Gerontol A Biol Sci Med Sci 64, 927-939, 2009b.

Fleg JL, O'Connor F, Gerstenblith G, Becker LC, Clulow J, Schulman SP, Lakatta EG. Impact of age on the cardiovascular response to dynamic upright exercise in healthy men and women. J Appl Physiol 78, 890-900, 1995.

Fleg JL, Morrell CH, Bos AG, Brant LJ, Talbot LA, Wright JG, Lakatta EG. Accelerated longitudinal decline of aerobic capacity in healthy older adults. Circulation 112, 674682, 2005.

Foster C. VO2max and training indices as determinants of competitive running performance. J Sports Sci 1, 13-22, 1983.

Fox EL, Bartels RL, Billings CE, Mathews DK, Bason R, Webb WM. Intensity and distance of interval training programs and changes in aerobic power. Med Sci Sports 5, 18-22, 1973.

Francescato MP, Cettolo V, di Prampero PE. Influence of phosphagen concentration on phosphocreatine breakdown kinetics. Data from human gastrocnemius muscle. J Appl Physiol 105, 158-164, 2008.

Garber CE, Blissmer B, Deschenes MR, Franklin BA, Lamonte MJ, Lee IM, Nieman DC, Swain DP. American College of Sports Medicine position stand. Quantity and quality of exercise for developing and maintaining cardiorespiratory, musculoskeletal, and neuromotor fitness in apparently healthy adults: guidance for prescribing exercise. Med Sci Sports Exerc 43, 1334-1359, 2011.

Garcin M, Vandewalle H, Monod H. A new rating scale of perceived exertion based on subjective estimation of exhaustion time: a preliminary study. Int J Sports Med 20, 40-43, 1999.

Gelfi C, Vigano A, Ripamonti M, Pontoglio A, Begum S, Pellegrino MA, Grassi B, Bottinelli R, Wait R, Cerretelli P. The human muscle proteome in aging. J Proteome Res 5, 1344-1353, 2006.

Gellish RL, Goslin BR, Olson RE, McDonald A, Russi GD, Moudgil VK. Longitudinal modeling of the relationship between age and maximal heart rate. Med Sci Sports Exerc 39, 822-829, 2007.

Giada F, Bertaglia E, De Piccoli B, Franceschi M, Sartori F, Raviele A, Pascotto P. Cardiovascular adaptations to endurance training and detraining in young and older athletes. Int J Cardiol 65, 149-155, 1998.

Gibala MJ, Little JP, Macdonald MJ, Hawley JA. Physiological adaptations to low volume, high-intensity interval training in health and disease. J Physiol 590, 10771084, 2012.

Gueguen N, Lefaucheur L, Herpin P. Relations entre fonctionnement mitochondrial et types contractiles des fibres musculaires. INRA Prod Anim 19, 265-278, 2006. Guzun R, Saks V. Application of the principles of systems biology and Wiener's cybernetics for analysis of regulation of energy fluxes in muscle cells in vivo. Int J Mol Sci 1, 982-1019, 2010.

Guzun R, Timohhina N, Tepp K, Monge C, Kaambre T, Sikk P, Kuznetsov AV, Pison C, Saks V. Regulation of respiration controlled by mitochondrial creatine kinase in permeabilized cardiac cells in situ. Importance of system level properties. Biochim Biophys Acta 1787, 1089-1105, 2009.

Hafstad AD, Boardman NT, Lund J, Hagve M, Khalid AM, Wisløff U, Larsen TS, Aasum E. High intensity interval training alters substrate utilization and reduces oxygen consumption in the heart. J Appl Physiol 111, 1235-1241, 2011.

Hagberg JM, Coyle EF, Carroll JE, Miller JM, Martin WH, Brooke MH. Exercise hyperventilation in patients with McArdle's disease. J Appl Physiol Respir Environ Exerc Physiol 52, 991-994, 1982.

Hagberg JM, Coyle EF. Physiological determinants of endurance performance as studied in competitive racewalkers. Med Sci Sports Exerc 15, 287-289, 1983.

Hampson DB, St Clair Gibson A, Lambert MI, Noakes TD. The influence of sensory cues on the perception of exertion during exercise and central regulation of exercise performance. Sports Med 31, 935-952, 2001.

Hawkins S, Wiswell R. Rate and mechanism of maximal oxygen consumption decline with aging: implications for exercise training. Sports Med 33, 877-888, 2003.

Heck H, Mader A, Hess G, Mücke S, Müller R, Hollmann W. Justification of the 4-mmol/l lactate threshold. Int J Sports Med 6, 117-130, 1985.

Helgerud J, Høydal K, Wang E, Karlsen T, Berg P, Bjerkaas M, Simonsen T, Helgesen C, Hjorth N, Bach R, Hoff J. Aerobic high-intensity intervals improve $\dot{V}O_2max$ more than moderate training. Med Sci Sports Exerc 39, 665-671, 2007.

Hermansen L, Stensvold I. Production and removal of lactate during exercise in man. Acta Physiol Scand 86, 191-201, 1972.

Hermansen L, Vaage O. Lactate disappearance and glycogen synthesis in human muscle after maximal exercise. Am J Physiol 233, E422-429, 1977.

Hill AV. Muscular movement in man. New York, Mc Graw-Hill, 104 p, 1927. Hill DW, Rowell AL. Running velocity at VO2max. Med Sci Sports Exerc 28, 114-119, 1996.

Hill DW, Williams CS, Burt SE. Responses to exercise at 92% and 100% of the velocity associated with VO2max. Int J Sports Med 18, 325-329, 1997.

Howald H. Effects of sport activities on the metabolism. [Article in German]. Schweiz Med Wochenschr 104, 1535-1538, 1974.

Howley ET, Bassett DR Jr, Welch HG. Criteria for maximal oxygen uptake: review and commentary. Med Sci Sports Exerc 27, 1292-1301, 1995.

Hughes EF, Turner SC, Brooks GA. Effects of glycogen depletion and pedaling speed on "anaerobic threshold." J Appl Physiol Respir Environ Exerc Physiol 52, 1598-1607, 1982.

Hughson R.L. Blood lactate concentration increases as a continuous function in progressive exercise. J. Appl. Physiol 62, 1975-1981, 1987.

Hunter GR1, McCarthy JP, Bamman MM. Effects of resistance training on older adults. Sports Med 34, 329-348, 2004.

Iaiche R, Toraa M, Friemel F. Evaluation de VO2max et de VMA en laboratoire et sur le terrain. Science et Sports 11, 91-95, 1996.

Ivy JL, Withers RT, Van Handel PJ, Elger DH, Costill DL. Muscle respiratory capacity and fiber type as determinants of the lactate threshold. J Appl Physiol Respir Environ Exerc Physiol 48, 523-527, 1980.

Jorfeldt L, Juhlin-Dannfelt A, Karlsson J. Lactate release in relation to tissue lactate in human skeletal muscle during exercise. J Appl Physiol Respir Environ Exerc Physiol 44, 350-352, 1978.

Kachouri M, Vandewalle H, Huet M, Thomaïdis M, Jousselin E, Monod, H. Is the time to exhaustion at maximal aerobic speed an index of aerobic endurance? Arch Int Physiol Biochem 104, 330-336, 1996a.

Kachouri M, Vandewalle H, Billat V, Huet M, Thomaïdis M, Jousselin E, Monod H. Critical velocity of continuous and intermittent running exercise. An example of the limits of the critical power concept. Eur J Appl Physiol Occup Physiol 73, 484-487, 1996b.

Kaczor JJ, Ziolkowski W, Antosiewicz J, Hac S, Tarnopolsky MA, Popinigis J. The effect of aging on anaerobic and aerobic enzyme activities in human skeletal muscle. J Gerontol A Biol Sci Med Sci 61, 339-344, 2006.

Karvonen J. Physiological follow-up of endurance runners. Report for the Finish Sport Foundation, Helsinki, 1983.

Kindermann W, Simon G, Keul J. The significance of the aerobic-anaerobic transition for the determination of workload intensities during endurance training. Eur J Appl Physiol Occup Physiol 42, 25-34, 1979.

Korzeniewski B, Zoladz JA. Biochemical background of the VO2 on-kinetics in skeletal muscles. J Physiol Sci 56, 1-12, 2006.

Kraus BJ, Brandon MP, Robinson RJ, Connerney MA, Hasselmo ME, Eichenbaum H. During Running in Place, Grid Cells Integrate Elapsed Time and Distance Run. Neuron 88, 578-589, 2015.

Kuipers H, Verstappen FT, Keize HA, Geurten P, VanKranenburg G. Variability of aerobic performance in the laboratory and its physiologic correlates. Int J Sports Med 6, 197-201, 1985.

Lacour JR, Candau R. Vitesse maximale aérobie et performance en course à pied. Science et Sports 5, 183-189, 1990.

Lacour JR, Montmayeur A, Dormois D, Gacon G, Padilla, S, Viale C. Validation de l'épreuve de mesure de la vitesse maximale aérobie (VMA) dans un groupe de coureurs de haut niveau. Science et Motricité 7, 3-8, 1989.

Lacour JR, Padilla-Magunacelaya S, Barthélémy JC, Dormois D. The energetics of middle-distance running. Eur J Appl Physiol Occup Physiol 60, 38-43, 1990.

Lacour JR, Padilla-Magunacelaya S, Chatard JC, Arsac, L, Barthélémy, JC. Assessment of running velocity at maximal oxygen uptake. Eur J Appl Physiol 62, 77-82, 1991.

LaFontaine TP, Londeree BR, Spath WK. The maximal steady state versus selected running events. Med Sci Sports Exerc 13, 190-193, 1981.

Larsen S, Nielsen J, Hansen CN, Nielsen LB, Wibrand F, Stride N, Schroder HD, Boushel R, Helge JW, Dela F, Hey-Mogensen M. Biomarkers of mitochondrial content in skeletal muscle of healthy young human subjects. J Physiol 590, 3349-3360, 2012.

Launay T, Momken I, Carreira S, Mougenot N, Zhou XL, De Koning L, Niel R, Riou B, Billat V, Besse S. Acceleration-based training : A new mode of training in senescent rats improving performance and left ventricular and muscle functions. Exp Gerontol 95, 71-76, 2017.

Lecarpentier Y1, Chemla D, Blanc FX, Pourny JC, Joseph T, Riou B, Coirault C. Mechanics, energetics, and crossbridge kinetics of rabbit diaphragm during congestive heart failure. FASEB J 12, 981-989, 1998.

Lechevalier JM, Vandewalle H, Chatard JC, Moreaux A, Gandrieux V, Besson F, Monod, H. Relationship between the 4 mmol running velocity, the time-distance relationship and the Léger-Boucher's test. Arch Int Physiol Biochem 97, 355-360, 1989.

Léger L, Boucher R. An indirect continuous running multistage field test: the Université de Montréal track test. Can J Appl Sport Sci 5, 77-84, 1980.

Léger L., Mercier D. Gross energy cost of horizontal treadmill and track running. Sports Med 1, 270-277, 1984.

Léger L, Gadoury C. Validity of the 20-m shuttle run test with 1 min stages to predict VO2max in adults. Can J Sport Sci 14, 21-26, 1989.

Léger L, Mercier D, Gauvin L. The relationship between %VO2max and running performance time. Sport and Elite Performers, Vol 3, Proceeding of 1984 Olympic Scientific Congress. Human Kinetics, Champaign IL, USA, 212 pages, 1986.

Léger LA, Mercier D, Gadoury C, Lambert J. The multistage 20 metre shuttle run test for aerobic fitness. J Sports Sci 6, 93-101, 1988.

Léger L, Ahmaidi S, Berthoin S, Cazorla G, Fargeas MA., Gerbeaux M, Lensel-Corbeil G, Prefaut, C. Estimation of the maximal aerobic speed from the maximal 20-m shuttle run test. Ped Exerc Sci 5, 438, 1993.

Lepers R, Cattagni T. Do older athletes reach limits in their performance during marathon running? Age 34, 773-781, 2012.

Leprêtre PM, Foster C, Koralsztein JP, Billat VL. Heart rate deflection point as a strategy to defend stroke volume during incremental exercise. J Appl Physiol 98, 16601665, 2005.

Londeree BR, Ames SA. Maximal steady state versus state of conditioning. Eur J Appl Physiol Occup Physiol 34, 269-278, 1975.

Lovell DI, Cuneo R, Gass GC. Strength training improves sub-maximum cardiovascular performance in older men. J Geriatr Phys Ther 32, 117-124, 2009.

MacDougall JD. The anaerobic threshold: its significance for the endurance athlete. Can J Appl Sport Sci 2, 137-140, 1977.

MacInnis MJ, Gibala MJ. Physiological adaptations to interval training and the role of exercise intensity. J Physiol 595, 2915-2930, 2017.

Mackworth NH. Vigilance. Adv Sci 53, 389-393, 1957.

Mader A, Heck H. A theory of the metabolic origin of "anaerobic threshold". Int J Sports Med 7 Suppl 1, 45-65, 1986.

Malek MH1, Hüttemann M, Lee I, Coburn JW. Similar skeletal muscle angiogenic and mitochondrial signaling following 8 weeks of endurance exercise in mice: discontinuous versus continuous training. Exp Physiol 98, 807-818, 2013.

Massicotte DR, Macnab RB. Cardiorespiratory adaptations to training at specified intensities in children. Med Sci Sports Exerc 6, 242-246, 1974.

McGuire DK, Levine BD, Williamson JW, Snell PG, Blomqvist CG, Saltin B, Mitchell JH. A 30-year follow-up of the Dallas Bedrest and Training Study: I. Effect of age on the cardiovascular response to exercise. Circulation 104, 1350-1357, 2001.

McMullan RC, Kelly SA, Hua K, et al. Long-term exercise in mice has sex-dependent benefits on body composition and metabolism during aging. Physiological Reports 4e13011, doi :10.14814/phy2.13011, 2016.

Medbø J, Mohn AC, Tabata I, Bahr R, Vaage O, Sejersted, OM. Anaerobic capacity determined by maximal accumulated O2 deficit. J Appl Physiol 64, 50-60, 1988.

Melin B, Jimenez C, Charpenet A, Pouzeratte N, Bittel J. Validation de deux tests de détermination de la vitesse maximale aérobie (VMA) sur le terrain. Science et Sports 11, 46-52, 1996.

Messonnier L, Denis C, Prieur F, Lacour JR. Are the effects of training on fat metabolism involved in the improvement of performance during high-intensity exercise ? Eur J Appl Physiol 94, 434-441, 2005.

Montmayeur A, Villaret M. Etude de la vitesse maximale aérobie derrière cycliste. Science et Motricité 10, 27-31, 1990.

Morgan DW, Baldini FD, Martin PE. Ten-kilometer performance and predicted velocity at VO2 max among well-trained male runners' threshold. Med Sci Sports Exerc 21, 78-83, 1989.

Myburgh KH, Viljoen A, Tereblanche S. Plasma lactate concentrations for self-selected maximal effort lasting 1 h. Med Sci Sports Exerc 33, 152-156, 2001.

Myers J, Prakash M, Froelicher V, Do D, Partington S, Atwood JE. Exercise capacity and mortality among men referred for exercise testing. N Engl J Med 346, 793-801, 2002.

Nagle F, Robinhold D, Howley E, Daniels J, Baptista G, Stoedefalke K. Lactic acid accumulation during running at submaximal aerobic demands. Med Sci Sports 2, 182186, 1970.

Nemutlu E, Zhang S, Gupta A, Juranic NO, Macura SI, Terzic A, Jahangir A, Dzeja

P. Dynamic phosphometabolomic profiling of human tissues and transgenic models by 18O-assisted ^{31}P NMR and mass spectrometry. Physiol Genomics 44, 386-402, 2012.

Niel R. Effets métaboliques et physiologiques d'un entraînement en accélération chez la souris âgée et effets de l'âge sur les capacités physiques de la souris déficiente à la créatine kinase. Thèse, Université d'Evry-Paris Saclay, 2017.

Niel R, Ayachi M, Mille-Hamard L, Le Moyec L, Savarin P, Clement MJ, Besse S, Launay T, Billat VL, Momken I. A new model of short acceleration-based training improves exercise performance in old mice. Scand J Med Sci Sports 27, 1576-1587, 2017.

Noakes TD. Time to move beyond a brainless exercise physiology: the evidence for complex regulation of human exercise performance. Appl Physiol Nutr Metab 36, 23-35, 2011.

Nybo L, Nielsen B. Perceived exertion is associated with an altered brain activity during exercise with progressive hyperthermia. J Appl Physiol 91, 2017-2023, 2001.

Ogawa T, Spina RJ, Martin WH 3rd, Kohrt WM, Schechtman KB, Holloszy JO, Ehsani AA. Effects of aging, sex, and physical training on cardiovascular responses to exercise. Circulation 86, 494-503, 1992.

Olivetti G, Melissari M, Capasso JM, Anversa P. Cardiomyopathy of the aging human heart. Myocyte loss and reactive cellular hypertrophy. Circ Res 68, 560-1568, 1991.

Padilla S, Bourdin M, Barthélémy JC, Lacour JR. Physiological correlates of middle-distance running performance. A comparative study between men and women. Eur J Appl Physiol Occup Physiol 65, 561-566, 1992.

Paoli A, Marcolin G, Zonin F, Neri M, Sivieri A, Pacelli QF. Exercising fasting or fed to enhance fat loss? Influence of food intake on respiratory ratio and excess post exercise oxygen consumption after a bout of endurance training. Int J Sport Nutr Exerc Metab 21, 48-54, 2011.

Pendergast D, Leibowitz R, Wilson D, Cerretelli P. The effect of preceding anaerobic exercise on aerobic and anaerobic work. Eur J Appl Physiol Occup Physiol 52, 29-35, 1983.

Péronnet F., Thibault G. Analyse physiologique de la performance en course à pied, révision du modèle hyperbolique. J Physiol (Paris) 82, 52-60, 1987.

Perry CG, Heigenhauser GJ, Bonen A, Spriet LL. High-intensity aerobic interval training increases fat and carbohydrate metabolic capacities in human skeletal muscle. Appl Physiol Nutr Metab 33, 1112-1123, 2008.

Perry CG, Kane DA, Herbst EA, Mukai K, Lark DS, Wright DC, Heigenhauser GJ, Neufer PD, Spriet LL, Holloway GP. Mitochondrial creatine kinase activity and phosphate shuttling are acutely regulated by exercise in human skeletal muscle. J Physiol 590, 5475-5486, 2012.

Petot H, Meilland R, Le Moyec L, Mille-Hamard L, Billat VL. A new incremental test for VO2max accurate measurement by increasing VO_2max plateau duration, allowing the investigation of its limiting factors. Eur J Appl Physiol 112, 2267-2276, 2012.

Pimentel AE, Gentile CL, Tanaka H, Seals DR, Gates PE. Greater rate of decline in maximal aerobic capacity with age in endurance-trained than in sedentary men. J Appl Physiol 94, 2406-2413, 2003.

Pires FO, Noakes TD, Lima-Silva AE, Bertuzzi R, Ugrinowitsch C, Lira FS, Kiss MA. Cardiopulmonary, blood metabolite and rating of perceived exertion responses to constant exercises performed at different intensities until exhaustion. Br J Sports Med 45, 1119-1125, 2011.

Pugh LG. Oxygen intake in track and treadmill running with observations on the effect of air resistance. J Physiol 207, 823-835, 1970.

Puype J, Van Proeyen K, Raymackers JM, Deldicque L, Hespel P. Sprint interval training in hypoxia stimulates glycolytic enzyme activity. Med Sci Sports Exerc 45, 21662174, 2013.

Reaburn P, Dascombe B. Anaerobic performance in master's athletes. Eur Rev Aging Phys Act 6, 39-53, 2009.

Rieu M, Ferry A, Martin MC, Duvallet A. Effect of previous supramaximal work on lacticaemia during supra-anaerobic threshold exercise. Eur J Appl Physiol Occup Physiol 61, 223-229, 1990.

Rodas G, Ventura JL, Cadefau JA, Cussó R, Parra J. A short training programme for the rapid improvement of both aerobic and anaerobic metabolism. Eur J Appl Physiol 82, 480-486, 2000.

Rossiter HB, Ward SA, Kowalchuk JM, Howe FA, Griffiths JR, Whipp BJ. Dynamic asymmetry of phosphocreatine concentration and O2 uptake between the on- and off-transients of moderate- and high-intensity exercise in humans. J Physiol 541, 9911002, 2002.

Rossiter HB, Howlett RA, Holcombe HH, Entin PL, Wagner HE, Wagner PD. Age is no barrier to muscle structural, biochemical and angiogenic adaptations to training up to 24 months in female rats. J Physiol 565, 993-1005, 2005.

Roy A, Sil PC. Tertiary butyl hydroperoxide induced oxidative damage in mice erythrocytes: Protection by taurine. Pathophysiology 19, 137-148, 2012.

Safdar A, Bourgeois JM, Ogborn DI, Little JP, Hettinga BP, Akhtar M, Thompson JE, Melov S, Mocellin NJ, Kujoth GC, Prolla TA, Tarnopolsky MA. Endurance exercise rescues progeroid aging and induces systemic mitochondrial rejuvenation in mtDNA mutator mice. Proc Natl Acad Sci 108, 4135-4140, 2011.

Saks VA, Kongas O, Vendelin M, Kay L. Role of the creatine/phosphocreatine system in the regulation of mitochondrial respiration. Acta Physiol Scand 168, 635-41, 2000.

Saks V, Favier R, Guzun R, Schlattner U, Wallimann T. Molecular system bioenergetics: regulation of substrate supply in response to heart energy demands. J Physiol 577, 769-77, 2006.

Saks V, Kaambre T, Guzun R, Anmann T, Sikk P, Schlattner U, Wallimann T, Aliev M, Vendelin M. The creatine kinase phosphor-transfer network: thermodynamic and kinetic considerations, the impact of the mitochondrial outer membrane and modelling approaches. Subcell Biochem 46, 27-65, 2007.

Sanada K, Kearns CF, Kojima K, Abe T. Peak oxygen uptake during running and arm cranking normalized to total and regional skeletal muscle mass measured by magnetic resonance imaging. Eur J Appl Physiol 93, 687-93, 2005.

Santos-Lozano A, Collado PS, Foster C, Lucia A, Garatachea N. Influence of sex and level on marathon pacing strategy. Insights from the New York City race. Int J Sports Med 35, 933-938, 2014. Scherrer J. La Fatigue. Que sais-je ? n°733, PUF, Paris, 1989.

Scherrer J., Monod H. Le travail musculaire local et la fatigue chez l'homme. J physiol (Paris) 52, 419-501, 1960.

Schlattner U, Tokarska-Schlattner M, Wallimann T. Mitochondrial creatine kinase in human health and disease. Biochim Biophys Acta 1762, 164-180, 2006.

Senefeld J, Joyner MJ, Stevens A, Hunter SK. Sex differences in elite swimming with advanced age are less than marathon running. Scand J Med Sci Sports 26, 17-28, 2016.

Serna VHA, Arango Vélez EF, Gómez Arias RD, Feito Y. Effects of a high-intensity interval training program versus a moderate-intensity continuous training program on maximal oxygen uptake and blood pressure in healthy adults: study protocol for a randomized controlled trial. Trials 17, 413, 2016.

Shephard RJ. A nomogram to calculate the oxygen-cost of running at slow speeds. J Sports Med Phys Fitness 9, 10-6, 1969.

Shephard RJ, Vandewalle H, Gil V, Bouhlel E, Monod H. Respiratory, muscular and overall perceptions of effort: the influence of hypoxia and muscle mass. Med Sci Sports Exerc 24, 556-567, 1992.

Shi X, Horn MK, Osterberg KL, Stofan JR, Zachwieja JJ, Horswill CA, Passe DH, Murray R. Gastrointestinal discomfort during intermittent high-intensity exercise: effect of carbohydrate-electrolyte beverage. Int J Sport Nutr Exerc Metab 14, 673-683, 2004.

Shih H, Lee B, Lee RJ, Boyle AJ. The aging heart and post-infarction left ventricular remodeling. J Am Coll Cardiol 57, 9-17, 2011.

Shimada K, Jong CJ, Takahashi K, Schaffer SW. Role of ROS Production and Turnover in the Antioxidant Activity of Taurine. Adv Exp Med Biol 803, 581-596, 2015.

Shiraev T, Barclay G. Evidence based exercise – clinical benefits of high intensity interval training. Aust Fam Physician 41, 960-962, 2012.

Siu PM, Donley DA, Bryner RW, Alway SE. Citrate synthase expression and enzyme activity after endurance training in cardiac and skeletal muscles. J Appl Physiol 94, 555-5560, 2003.

Sjödin B, Jacobs I. Onset of blood lactate accumulation and marathon running performance. Int J Sports Med 2, 23-26, 1981.

Sjödin B, Jacobs I, Svedenhag J. Changes in onset of blood lactate accumulation (OBLA) and muscle enzymes after training at OBLA. Eur J Appl Physiol Occup Physiol 49, 45-57, 1982.

Skinner JS, McLellan TM. The transition from aerobic to anaerobic metabolism. Res Q Exerc Sport 51, 234-48, 1980.

Snyder AC, Jeukendrup AE, Hesselink MK, Kuipers H, Foster C. A physiological/psychological indicator of over-reaching during intensive training. Int J Sports Med 14, 29-32, 1993.

Spina RJ, Chi MM, Hopkins MG, Nemeth PM, Lowry OH, Holloszy JO. Mitochondrial enzymes increase in muscle in response to 7-10 days of cycle exercise. J Appl Physiol 80, 2250-2254, 1996.

St Clair Gibson A, Lambert ML, Noakes TD. Neural control of force output during maximal and submaximal exercise. Sports Med 31, 637-650, 2001.

Stegmann H, Kindermann W. Comparison of prolonged exercise tests at the individual anaerobic threshold and the fixed anaerobic threshold of 4 mmol.l-1.lactate. Int J Sports Med 3, 105-110, 1982.

Stephens FB, Galloway SD. Carnitine and fat oxidation. Nestle Nutr Inst Workshop Ser 76, 13-23, 2013.

Stoudemire NM, Wideman L, Pass KA, McGinnes CL, Gaesser GA, Weltman A. The validity of regulating blood lactate concentration during running by ratings of perceived exertion. Med Sci Sports Exerc 28, 490-495, 1996.

Swain DP. Moderate or vigorous intensity exercise: which is better for improving aerobic fitness? Prev Cardiol 8, 55-58, 2005.

Tabata I, Nishimura K, Kouzaki M, Hirai Y, Ogita F, Miyachi M, Yamamoto K. Effects of moderate-intensity endurance and high-intensity intermittent training on anaerobic capacity and VO2max. Med Sci Sports Exerc 28, 1327-1330, 1996.

Tanaka H, Seals DR. Endurance exercise performance in Masters athletes: age-associated changes and underlying physiological mechanisms. J Physiol 586, 55-63, 2008.

Tepp K, Timohhina N, Puurand M, Klepinin A, Chekulayev V, Shevchuk I, Kaambre T. Bioenergetics of the aging heart and skeletal muscles: Modern concepts and controversies. Ageing Res Rev 28, 1-14, 2016.

Timohhina N, Guzun R, Tepp K, Monge C, Varikmaa M, Vija H, Sikk P, Kaambre T, Sackett D, Saks V. Direct measurement of energy fluxes from mitochondria into cytoplasm in permeabilized cardiac cells in situ: some evidence for Mitochondrial Interactosome. J Bioenerg Biomembr 41, 259-275, 2009.

Tintignac LA, Brenner HR, Rüegg MA. Mechanisms Regulating Neuromuscular Junction Development and Function and Causes of Muscle Wasting. Physiol Rev 95, 809852, 2015.

Tuikkala P, Hartikainen S, Korhonen M, Lavikainen P, Kettunen R, Sulkava R, Enlund H. Serum total cholesterol levels and all-cause mortality in a home-dwelling elderly population: a six-year follow-up. Scand J Prim Health Care, 121-127, 2010.

Van Loon LJ, Greenhaff PL, Constantin-Teodosiu D, Saris WH, Wagenmakers AJ. The effects of increasing exercise intensity on muscle fuel utilization in humans. J Physiol 536, 295-304, 2001.

Ventura-Clapier R, De Sousa E, Veksler V. Metabolic myopathy in heart failure. News Physiol Sci 17, 191-196, 2002.

Ventura-Clapier R. Créatine kinases et transferts d'énergie dans le myocyte cardiaque. médecine/sciences 14, 1017-1024, 1998.

Wall BT, Stephens FB, Constantin-Teodosiu D, Marimuthu K, Macdonald IA, Greenhaff PL. Chronic oral ingestion of L-carnitine and carbohydrate increases muscle carnitine content and alters muscle fuel metabolism during exercise in humans. J Physiol 589, 963–973, 2011.

Wasserman K. The anaerobic threshold measurement in exercise testing. Clin Chest Med 5, 77-88, 1984.

Wasserman K., Mc Ilroy M.B. Detecting the threshold of anaerobic metabolism in cardiac patients during exercise. Am. J. Cardiol 14, 844-852, 1964.

Wasserman K, Whipp BJ, Koyl SN, Beaver WL. Anaerobic threshold and respiratory gas exchange during exercise. J Appl Physiol 35, 236-243, 1973.

Whipp BJ, Wasserman K. Oxygen uptake kinetics for various intensities of constant load work. J Appl Physiol 33, 351-356, 1972. Whipp BJ, Ward SA. Will women soon outrun men? Nature 2355, 25, 1992.

White M, Roden R, Minobe W, Khan MF, Larrabee P, Wollmering M, Port JD,

Anderson F, Campbell D, Feldman AM. Age-related changes in beta-adrenergic neuroeffector systems in the human heart. Circulation 90, 1225-1238, 1994.

Wilson TM, Tanaka H. Meta-analysis of the age-associated decline in maximal aerobic capacity in men: relation to training status. Am J Physiol Heart Circ Physiol 278, H829834, 2000.

Witard OC, McGlory C, Hamilton DL, Phillips SM. Growing older with health and vitality: a nexus of physical activity, exercise and nutrition. Biogerontology 17, 529546, 2016.

Yoshida T. Effect of exercise duration during incremental exercise on the determination of anaerobic threshold and the onset of blood lactate accumulation. Eur J Appl Physiol Occup Physiol 53, 196-199, 1984.

Żoładź JA, Korzeniewski B. Physiological background of the change point in V˙O2 and the slow component of oxygen uptake kinetics. J Physiol Pharmacol 52, 167-184, 2001.

Zoll J, Sanchez H, N'Guessan B, Ribera F, Lampert E, Bigard X, Serrurier B, Fortin D, Geny B, Veksler V, Ventura-Clapier R, Mettauer B. Physical activity changes the regulation of mitochondrial respiration in human skeletal muscle. J Physiol 543, 191-200, 2002.

THE SCIENCE OF THE MARATHON AND THE ART OF VARIABLE PACE RUNNING

This book was written by Veronique Billat, Ph.D. (University of Paris-Saclay) and Johnathan Edwards, M.D. (University of Paris-Saclay).

www.ingramcontent.com/pod-product-compliance
Lightning Source LLC
Chambersburg PA
CBHW081354290426
44110CB00018B/2377